Making a Balanced Vaccination Decision

A Guide for Parents

Oliver Müller
4th Edition

Content

Introduction

The information presented in this book was first published in form of an app, until Apple unilaterally removed it from its AppStore in December 2014. Over the phone Apple told me that the reason was that medical information should come from a medical institution only. But they also admitted that they would not demand the same of any other apps in the medical category.

Unfortunately there are those who believe that any information which does not portray vaccinations as completely safe and completely effective should be censored. But science is never as simple as newspaper headlines and I have yet to find a single regulatory assessment report or even any manufacturer's information which is as unequivocally pro-vaccine as the fanatics who haunt the internet, trolling social media and complaining to Apple about the content of apps. No medication, including vaccines, should be beyond question. If they are, they become a matter of religion and not science.

The information contained in this book is based on the Vaccination Information Portal mobile app (still available for Android) but has since been updated and added to. My sources are almost exclusively one of the following: National Health Service, Office of National Statistics, Health Protection Agency (all UK), Federal Drug Administration, Center for Disease Control and Prevention (both US), vaccine manufacturers and studies published in peer-reviewed medical journals and referenced on PubMed. Some other sources are used where appropriate and as referenced.

Although much of the content is UK-based, there is no reason why parents would not benefit from it anywhere in the world. England has one of the longest-running record on infectious diseases and much of the information is transferable to other countries. The main difference is that many more vaccines are used in the USA but most of the diseases vaccinated against all over the world are covered here.

If you are a parent looking for balanced and referenced information on routine childhood vaccinations which is sourced from official sources but nevertheless not afraid to be critical of vaccinations, then this book is for you.

Note on current edition

In this 4th edition I have added a chapter for Bexsero, the new Men B vaccine. I have also amended the chapter on meningococcal infections and the chapter Whom to Believe.

Although an alternative vaccine to Pediacel was introduced in the UK in 2014 (Infanrix-IPV-Hib), very little useful information is currently in the public domain and I have therefore not included it at this time. The manufacturer's package insert is available but didn't prove very useful. I was after the public assessment report which can normally be found on one of the regulators' websites. But the European Medicines Agency referred me to the UK regulator (MHRA) and they in turn told me there was no such report because the vaccine was licensed before the law required these reports to be compiled and published.

I have assumed that not all readers will read the book cover to cover and that many will simply look up the disease or vaccine they are interested in at that time. For this reason there is some repetition among some of the vaccine chapters and any reader who is reading through the entire book will notice these.

General Information

General Information about Vaccine Efficacy

Assessing the efficacy of a vaccine usually starts with testing its *immunogenicity*, which is the same as saying we measure the body's antibody response to the vaccines. If there are enough antibodies, then this is usually equated with immunity, even though it has long been proved that a high level of antibodies does not mean a person cannot get ill. [1,2,3,4,5,6] In fact, antibody levels have been shown to tell us very little about the likelihood of a person becoming ill. The immune system is only partly understood and blood antibodies are only a small part of it.

In addition to this, vaccines sometimes also undergo a clinical trial where a large number of people are vaccinated and the researchers look at whether these people get ill less often than a "placebo" group. If they do, the vaccine is also considered *efficacious*. Here we have a more realistic view of whether a vaccine works but it is still important to remember that these studies are carried out by the manufacturers of the vaccines and that they control how the data is handled. In addition, the placebo is, in many cases, another vaccine.

Sometimes, so-called non-inferiority studies are used to show that a vaccine is at least as good as one which is already in use, once again based on immunogenicity.

Effectiveness, as opposed to efficacy, of a vaccine is usually assessed retrospectively by looking at whether a vaccine has made a positive impact in real life. Sometimes this is easy. If almost every student in a school was fully vaccinated and the school still suffered an outbreak, then the vaccine was not effective. But most of the time it is highly complicated, as data needs to be adjusted for so-called confounding factors. For example care home residents may be more likely to have a vaccine but are also more likely to get ill due to age and frailty. The problem here is that by the time the data has been adjusted, it can be made to say almost anything.
Regardless of the detail of any study, manufacturers will of course publish the positive ones and delay or bury those coming out negative. A study published in the BMJ in 2014 found that only around half of clinical trial get published after completion. Those that are published report a positive result in 98% of cases. Yet non-manufacturer-funded trials were over 4 times more likely to report negative results. [7]

Most of the scientific material available also shows that vaccine-induced "immunity" wears off, sometimes quickly, sometimes over many years. This has led to a number of problems, which are discussed in the relevant chapters. This "waning immunity" can mean a choice of life-long boosters or allowing a child to go through the disease, thereby acquiring true life-long "natural" immunity.

References

1. J Infect Dis. 2009 May 15;199(10):1457-60
2. Vaccine. 2007 Jun 11;25(24):4665-70
3. J Exp Med. 1969 Jun 1;129(6):1307-26
4. Am J Infect Control. 1992 Dec;20(6):319-25
5. Infect Control Hosp Epidemiol. 1990 Sep;11(9):473-8
6. Vaccine. 2008 Apr 16;26(17):2111-8
7. BMJ 2014;348:g3058

General Information about Vaccine Safety

When it comes to the safety of vaccines, it has to be remembered that:

a) side-effects (also called adverse reactions or adverse events) are normally compared to other vaccines during trial, and rarely to a true placebo

b) many studies only consider adverse reaction to be caused by the vaccine if they happen within a few days of the vaccine being given

c) long-term safety is rarely studied and difficult to determine

d) the long-term and cumulative effect of non-active ingredients such as mercury and aluminium adjuvants is little understood and seldom studied

e) whether or not vaccines are contributing to or even causing the epidemic we are seeing of autism is simply not known

f) vaccine damage is difficult to determine and adverse events are widely under-reported, with estimates ranging from only 1% – 10% of actual events being reported

g) heart-rendering stories of vaccine-damaged children found on the internet show that vaccines are not always safe but do not help assess the likelihood of such damage happening to your child

h) parents are advised to use all the information available here and elsewhere in order to make an informed decision.

Whom to Believe

When making vaccination decisions, parents will wonder whose information can be trusted. It should be remembered that:

- Vaccine manufacturer GlaxoSmithKline was fined a record $3bn in July 2012 for criminal behaviour, including withholding safety data
- Vaccine manufacturer Pfizer was fined $1.3bn ($2.3bn if costs are included) in 2009 for being a repeat offender in off-label marketing (selling drugs for conditions they aren't approved for); there were 3 previous cases.
- Vaccine manufacturer AstraZeneca was fined $355m in 2003 for a 3-year long Medicare fraud and settled claims without admitting liability, that it had bribed doctors. In 2010 it settled another $520m without admitting the charges, again for illegal marketing and illegal kick-backs to doctors. Further cases are too numerous to mention here.
- Vaccine manufacturer Merck has had to pay several billion dollars over recent years in criminal fines and to settle civil law suits over its illegal marketing of Vioxx.
- Vaccine manufacturer Wyeth (owned by Pfizer) was made to pay $490m in criminal and civil matters relating to illegal off-label marketing.
- Vaccine manufacturer Novartis agreed to pay $422m in fines and civil liabilities related to off-label marketing and paying kick-backs to doctors.
- Vaccine manufacturer Baxter has a multitude of smaller fines under its belt for various offences in the US, still amounting to many millions.

Doctors in the UK get paid for reaching certain levels of vaccination coverage.

These are 70% and 90% of their patients of the appropriate age and reaching these targets entitles them to the "lower" or "higher payments" respectively. The "bonus" payment is a fairly complicated calculation and varies with patient numbers but it certainly makes a difference of thousands of pounds to each practice.
This does not mean that GPs and/or their staff are dishonest or in it for the money. Most of them consider the issue of vaccination safety and effectiveness as settled and have few concerns over them. They have no time to do in-depth research and feel that they have to trust the NHS, government sources, the manufacturers or the regulators that are meant to oversee the manufacturers. But with this taken into account, parents do get pressured at times and the influence of bonus payments cannot be disregarded, especially if medical staff believe that a parent is refusing for no good reason. Medical staff should not be considered as necessarily being better informed about vaccinations than parents.

Government/regulators/independent research

There is now no clear boundary between industry financial interests and government agencies or departments. Increasingly the latter rely on "advisors" who come from industry and who retain financial interests in the pharmaceutical industry. They also rely on industry data and research and due to the lack of central funding for research, there is now only very little research done which is wholly independent of industry funding. Considering the amount of information which comes straight from vaccine manufacturers and the limited funding available for officials to examine these, parents are advised not to use so called "official" sources as their only source of information.

Internet and especially "anti-vaccination" websites

On the internet it is easy to spread rumours and repeat information which was stated somewhere, without checking the source or veracity. Parents may wish to read such information as a means of balancing the information given by "official" sources, bearing in mind that it may be inaccurate. However, it should also be noted that the individuals behind such websites do not stand to make any money from them and are normally investing much time and money in spreading the "truth" they believe in. This absence of monetary interest has to be taken into account when deciding whom to believe. It should also be noted that, as far as inaccuracies are concerned, I have also found a lot of these on "official" websites. Evidence offered by websites on the internet, even if anecdotal, should therefore not necessarily be seen as less valid.

Studies published in peer-reviewed medical journals

While for many of us this appears to be the ultimate source for reliable information, here too we need to be cautious. It never seems to get much publicity in the media but numerous current and former editors of medical journals have spoken out about the flawed peer-review process and have criticised their own industry as well as the pharmaceutical companies.

Dr Marcia Angell – former editor in chief of The New England Journal of Medicine has written about The Truth about the Drug Companies [1], Your Dangerous Drug Store [2] and Drug Companies & Doctors: A Story of Corruption [3] In the latter she states, "It is simply no longer possible to believe much of the clinical research that is published, or to rely on the judgment of trusted physicians or authoritative medical guidelines. I take no pleasure in this conclusion, which I reached slowly and reluctantly over my two decades as an editor of The New England Journal of Medicine."

Richard Smith – former editor (for 25 years) of the British Medical Journal and for 13 years of the BMJ Publishing Group has written about Medical journals and pharmaceutical companies: uneasy bedfellows [4], Medical Journals Are an Extension of the Marketing Arm of Pharmaceutical Companies [5], Peer review: a flawed process at the heart of science and journals [6], Should scientific fraud be a criminal offence? [7] and Revealed: how drug firms 'hoodwink' medical journals [8].
In [7] he states, "…research misconduct is common, terrifyingly common.
What is also highly unsatisfactory is how hundreds of studies (and probably many more) that are fraudulent remain in the scientific literature without any signal that they are inventions. I've been involved closely with two fraudulent researchers who between them have generated more than a hundred studies that are not retracted. Science is failing in its duty to the public.

Fraudsters escape because of the incompetence of the institutions, whereas investigation and collection of admissible evidence is the daily job of the police.
It's time, sadly, to criminalise research fraud."

And in [8] it is stated that, "Dr Richard Smith, editor of the British Journal of Medicine, admitted ghostwriting was a 'very big problem'. 'We are being hoodwinked by the drug companies. The articles come in with doctors' names on them and we often find some of them have little or no idea about what they have written,' he said."

Richard Horton – Editor of The Lancet has warned about The Dawn of McScience [9], in which he states, "Journals have devolved into information-laundering operations for the pharmaceutical industry."
Further, in the Lancet he has stated:
"The case against science is straightforward: much of the scientific literature, perhaps half, may simply be untrue. Afflicted by studies with small sample sizes, tiny effects, invalid exploratory analyses, and flagrant conflicts of interest, together with an obsession for pursuing fashionable trends of dubious importance, science has taken a turn towards darkness.
The apparent endemicity of bad research behaviour is alarming. In their quest for telling a compelling story, scientists too often sculpt data to fit their preferred theory of the world.
Journal editors deserve their fair share of criticism too. We aid and abet the worst behaviours. Our love of "significance" pollutes the literature with many a statistical fairy-tale.
Journals are not the only miscreants. Universities are in a perpetual struggle for money and talent, endpoints that foster reductive metrics, such as high-impact publication. National assessment procedures, such as the Research Excellence Framework, incentivise bad practices. And individual scientists, including their most senior leaders, do little to alter a research culture that occasionally veers close to misconduct." [10]

Drummond Rennie – former Deputy Editor of the New England Journal of Medicine and Journal of the American Medical Association (JAMA) wrote in Health Services Research [11]:
"It has been clear for at least two decades that, when clinical researchers have a financial stake in the results, it opens the door to a pervasive distortion of science. When a drug company sponsors a trial, the company employees usually select the drug tested, its dose, and the comparison drug. Company employees design the trial, often to produce the result they desire rather than to answer a scientific question. They have a powerful and fateful role in managing the trial, sometimes stopping it for reasons unrelated to science and despite any commitment to the trial participants. They may even suppress the results completely. ... In addition, they collect and analyze the data, and write up the report. In other settings, companies may "ghost-write" favorable meta-analyses of clinical studies. Only after the design, methods, and results are completed may the academic "authors" be selected and paid to have their names on the byline, thus joining in all but name the marketing arm of the sponsor. And authors frequently ignore the requests of editors to disclose their financial ties.

"For journals publishing reports directly applicable to the care of patients,...the distorting effect of money represents by far the single biggest challenge to the system's integrity. ... the Federal Drug Administration (FDA) has been emasculated. As a major new stream of funding for the FDA's critical roles of oversight and protection of the public's safety and health, the FDA has, since 1992, charged a pernicious user fee, which requires that companies seeking FDA approval pay the FDA to evaluate their drug applications. Congress has continued to reauthorize the relevant act. Predictably, this has had the effect of guaranteeing that the FDA, set up to protect the public, ends up beholden for its operating budget to the very industry the agency is supposed to regulate."

In Annals of Internal Medicine he wrote:
"The main point of the seeding trial is not to get high-quality scientific information: It is to change the prescribing habits of large numbers of physicians. A secondary purpose is to transform physicians into advocates for the sponsor's drug. The company flatters a physician by selecting him because he is "an opinion leader" and incorporates him in the research team with the title of "investigator." Then, it pays him good money: a consulting fee to advise the company on the drug's use and another fee for each patient he enrols. The physician becomes invested in the drug's future and praises its good features to patients and colleagues. Unwittingly, the physician joins the sponsor's marketing team. Why do companies pursue this expensive tactic? Because it works." [12]

These quotes come straight from the editors of the most prestigious journals in the world and can therefore hardly be ignored.

References

1. The New York Review of Books, July 2004
2. The New York Review of Books, June 2006
3. The New York Review of Books, January 2009
4. BMJ 2003;326:1202
5. PLoS Med 2(5): e138
6. J R Soc Med. 2006 Apr; 99(4): 178–182.
7. BMJ blog at http://blogs.bmj.com/bmj/2013/12/09/richard-smith-should-scientific-fraud-be-a-criminal-offence/
8. The Guardian website, December 2003, http://www.theguardian.com/society/2003/dec/07/health.businessofresearch
9. The New York Review of Books, March 2004
10. The Lancet Vol 385 April 11, 2015
11. Health Serv Res. 2010 Jun; 45(3): 885–896
12. Ann Intern Med. 2008;149(4):279-280

Herd Immunity

The concept of herd immunity should not be part of any vaccination decision. Herd immunity is a theory that says that if a certain percentage of the population is fully vaccinated against a disease, the disease cannot spread even among the unvaccinated and will therefore be eradicated. There is no scientific foundation to this idea. It started off with an arbitrary figure of 55% of the population and was incrementally increased over time to the current 95% or 98%. These figures are purely arbitrary and were changed whenever the previous percentage proved to be wrong. In one study, outbreaks of measles were found to have occurred even in populations with up to 99.8% vaccination rate. [1]

Even just a quick look at the historical charts in this book will show that vaccine-induced herd immunity cannot possibly exist. Otherwise, how could diseases have fallen by 99% before the vaccines were even introduced?

Further, as vaccinated people can pass on the disease against which they have been vaccinated, either through "shedding" from a live vaccine or because they became ill despite being vaccinated, it is even more illogical that a certain vaccination coverage could arrest the spread of disease and protect the unvaccinated. And finally, as no vaccine really imparts life-long immunity, any calculation of "vaccine-coverage" as a percentage of the population does not tell us anything about the level of protection.

By the time the required coverage thought to produce herd immunity had reached 95% (or similar, depending on the disease and on the source quoted), the whole concept had become meaningless and should have been abandoned there and then.

Unfortunately I have found numerous studies that use herd immunity to explain why incidents of a disease fell in the unvaccinated as much as in the vaccinated or why there is no large-scale outbreak in age-groups where vaccines are found to be the least effective. The correct conclusion would have been that the vaccine didn't make a difference in that particular case.

References

1. Arch Intern Med. 1994 Aug 22;154(16):1815-20

Diseases

Diphtheria

Diphtheria is a highly contagious bacterial infection caused by Corynebacterium diphtheriae, or more precisely by toxins produced by this bacterium. It mainly affects the throat or the nose. It is spread through the droplets in coughs and sneezes and can range from a mild illness to one which is life-threatening.

The risk of contracting diphtheria in the UK is very low. Statistics published by the Health Protection Agency show a sharp reduction in reported cases following the start of the vaccination campaign in 1941. [1] Such data can be questioned based on under-reporting or refusal by doctors to diagnose a disease for which a patient has been vaccinated. This is less likely with mortality figures. But these too show a clear reduction in cases after the introduction of the vaccine. How much the vaccine contributed to the decline of deaths from diphtheria, readers can decide for themselves from the following graph.

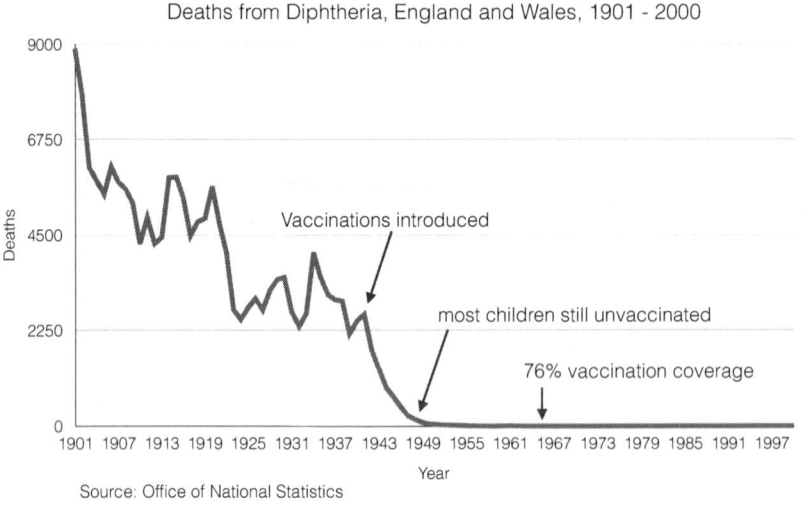

Deaths from Diphtheria, England and Wales, 1901 - 2000

Source: Office of National Statistics

There are now virtually no cases of diphtheria in the UK year on year. Is this due to ongoing vaccinations? Coverage levels are the same to other infectious diseases against which we vaccinate and these have not disappeared entirely. What about other countries?

The NHS website points to the 1990s epidemic in countries that had recently broken away from the former Soviet Union and claims that this was due to fewer children receiving the vaccines. In fact the disease mainly affected vaccinated adults. This epidemic was studied with great interest at the time particularly *because* of the high level of vaccination among the population. [2] The true cause was a collapse in living standards (poverty, reduced medical and social care, increased drug consumption) which also caused outbreaks of other diseases, such as hepatitis, measles, typhus and cholera.

The threat of diphtheria returning to the UK, therefore, seems more likely to hinge on living standards than vaccinations. As with all vaccines, plenty of studies say that the diphtheria vaccine is very effective, normally measured by antibody response. It is rare that such studies are independent of the manufacturer or their funding. If a vaccine causes antibodies to be produced, this is called immunogenicity. It doesn't guarantee immunity.

The immunogenicity caused by the vaccine reduces over time. A year 2000 study administered booster vaccines for diphtheria and monitored immunogenicity. [3] The booster did not work for 18% of cases and after 1 year, 7% of all subjects had lost the required antibody count again. Another study found 70% of people who had their last vaccination more than 10 years ago were "unprotected". Even worse, during a study in the Baltic states, the change in immunogenicity after a booster vaccine was negligible. [4] After 1-2 months the booster had only managed to raise the percentage of people with a "protective" antibody count from 60% to 80%. Far from the very high effectiveness which the vaccine is normally credited with.

The studies don't always agree on the detail, but normally they agree on the necessity for life-long boosters to keep the antibody count up. [6]

Parents may wonder if this is worth it, considering the almost zero risk in the UK. No one has died from Diphtheria in the UK in over 20 years and there were only 5 mortalities in the last 40 years.

In 1993 a report on an outbreak in 1989 in South Africa raised concerns about the vaccine having reduced the level of natural immunity to such an extent, that an outbreak was made possible. [5] Other studies too warn of the reduced natural immunity from vaccination programmes.

During an "outbreak" in Florida in 1969, 11 cases of diphtheria with 3 deaths were reported. "All patients resided in a predominantly black, low socioeconomic community", says the report. None of them had been vaccinated but neither had the many close contacts who were also carrying the same toxigenic bacterium and who were not showing any symptoms.[7]

Considering that not even the CDC considers anyone vaccinated if the person had their last diphtheria booster more than 10 years ago [8], most of us should not be "protected" from vaccinations and therefore it cannot be vaccinations that are keeping us safe from diphtheria.

The vaccines used against diphtheria in the UK are Pediacel, Infanrix-IPV, Repevax, and Revaxis.

References

1. Protecting the health of the Nation's children: the benefit of vaccines – Health Protection Agency
2. CDC MMWR Weekly Nov 05, 1993
3. Wien Med Wochenschr. 2000;150(22):435-9
4. J Infect Dis. 2000 Feb;181 Suppl 1:S213-9
5. Ann Trop Paediatr. 1993;13(1):13-9
6. Eur J Epidemiol. 1995 Feb;11(1):107-17
7. South Med J. 1976 Jun;69(6):759-61, 763
8. Am J Public Health. 1998 May; 88(5): 787–791

Flu

Flu (influenza) is a viral infection which everyone knows about because everyone has had it at various stages in their lives. In the UK a nasal flu vaccine is offered from 2-3 years of age and is intended to be continuously offered every year up to the age of 16.

The NHS says the nasal flu vaccine is even more effective than the injected vaccine and has fewer side-effects. Its website continues "your child is less likely to become ill if they come into contact with the flu virus".[1]

Leaving the matter of natural vs vaccine-induced immunity aside for now, how effective is the vaccine?

A study published in 1999 divided 4561 US citizens into two groups (nasal flu vaccine and placebo) and observed outcomes over one flu season (winter) in terms of "febrile illness", meaning illness which produced fever. Both groups were equally likely to get ill, although the vaccinated group was said to get ill less severely. [2] They found that the strain of influenza virus which was circulating at the time was a poor match to the the vaccine strain, which also highlights the practical, real-life problem of vaccinating against a constantly mutating virus.

A review of various trials (involving a total of 70,000 adults) published in 2010 found very little evidence that the flu vaccine prevented flu in adults, even though almost half of the studies included in the review were industry funded. The authors also noted that "Studies funded from public sources were significantly less likely to report conclusions favorable to the vaccines." [3] In the case of children, the same researchers found that six children under the age of six need to be vaccinated with live attenuated vaccine to prevent one case of influenza (infection and symptoms)." The say they could find "no usable data for those aged two years or younger" and that "Inactivated vaccines in children aged two years or younger are not significantly more efficacious than placebo." Here, too, industry-funded publications were included. The researchers conclude "The review showed that reliable evidence on influenza vaccines is thin but there is evidence of widespread manipulation of conclusions and spurious notoriety of the studies."

One meta-analysis published in 2012 found the intranasal flu vaccine highly effective in children aged 2-17, but as this analysis was, in fact, carried out by the manufacturer of the Fluenz vaccine, it has to be viewed with a fair amount of scepticism. [4]

A small randomised trial in Hong Kong found no significant difference [7] but various other studies found moderate effectiveness in protecting children. [5,6,0].

I was interested to read the study "Seasonal Influenza Vaccine Effectiveness" by the National Institute for Health Research. The study authors conclude that the tested vaccines were overall 57% effective but the raw data shows that those vaccinated were significantly more likely to require medical care or hospitalisation for related illnesses, as well as to die from related illnesses. I accept that some adjustment is needed to raw data (for example old and frail care home residents may be more likely to be vaccinated) but in the process of adjustment, almost any outcome can be reached and the results will be unreliable at best.

In March 2014 a study found that fully vaccinated children were 74% less likely to be admitted to intensive care with flu-related conditions. [9] Unfortunately there were only 44 cases included in the study, which was due to the rarity of flu becoming that serious. They also couldn't confirm the vaccination status of children in the control group and had to rely on what parents said/ remembered. Only those children who had had 2 doses of nasal flu vaccine were considered vaccinated in this US study. In the UK we use 1 dose. The study found no protective effect from one dose but considering its many flaws, it cannot really support any of its authors conclusions in any case.

A EuroSurveillance Study led by Public Health England and published in June 2014, examined the impact of flu vaccinations in primary school aged children during the 2013/14 flu season. It found little to no benefit. [10]
Another EuroSurveillance study, likewise led by Public Health England calculated Vaccine Effectiveness for the 2012/13 season at between 35% and 51% despite already having excluded one third of subjects from the analysis for reasons such as having been vaccinated too recently. [11]

Meanwhile recent studies in Australia calculated vaccine effectiveness at 13-15% for influenza A and 53% for influenza B, and in New Zealand at 0% (more vaccinated people got flu than non-vaccinated controls. [12,13]

References

1.   NHS Website January 2014
2.   JAMA. 1999 Jul 14;282(2):137-44
3.   Cochrane Database Syst Rev. 2010 Jul 7;(7):CD001269
4.   Vaccine. 2012 Jan 20;30(5):886-92
5.   Pediatr Infect Dis J. 2009 May;28(5):365-71
6.   Clin Ther. 2009 Oct;31(10):2140-7
7.   Vaccine. 2013 Apr 8;31(15):1937-43
8.   Pediatrics. 2007 Sep;120(3):e553-64
9.   J Infect Dis. (2014)
10.   Eurosurveillance, Volume 19, Issue 22, 05 June 2014
11.   Eurosurveillance, Volume 19, Issue 27, 10 July 2014
12.   Med J Aust. 2014 Jul 21;201(2):109-11
13.   N Z Med J. 2014 Jul 18;127(1398):12-8

Hib

Hib (Haemophilus influenzae type b) is a bacterial infection and it can cause a variety of symptoms, from mild coughs to meningitis, arthritis and pneumonia. The more serious infections are caused by the encapsulated form of which there are six types, types A-F. The vaccine is for type B, as this type most commonly causes invasive infections.

Hib mainly affects adults with underlying conditions according to the NHS, though ONS data shows that on average 0-2 children die of it per year. The risk is low but Hib meningitis is a possibility, of which there are 20-30 cases per year.

The Health Protection Agency says

> "After Hib vaccine was introduced marked reductions were observed in the number of cases of Hib disease in children under five years of age. *Disease rates also fell in older children and adults who had not been immunised* because the number of children carrying Hib bacteria, and therefore able to infect other people, fell."[2] (my italics)

So the disease rate fell in both the vaccinated and unvaccinated and the HPA puts it down to a herd immunity effect.

But we know from plenty of anecdotal evidence that doctors are much less likely to diagnose a disease for which a child has been vaccinated.
A study of children in the West Midlands published in the British Medical Journal in 2000 compared active and passive surveillance data for Hib infections before and after the vaccine was introduced. [1] They found significant under-reporting in just that age group that was supposed to be protected by the newly introduced vaccine, supporting the suspicion that because they had the vaccine, these children's cases were not reported. However, the difference, though significant at 23%, does not entirely explain the fall in reported cases.

Parents considering their vaccination decision might therefore assume that the vaccine does have a protective effect (56.7% effectiveness according to the HPA), provided that the simultaneous reduction in unvaccinated children is indeed due to some sort of herd immunity caused by the vaccine. One could equally argue the vaccine made no difference, as cases fell equally in the vaccinated and unvaccinated populations. A herd effect is difficult to believe with the low initial vaccination coverage. Unfortunately the data gets more confusing when we consider that the Health Protection Agency has found that Hib infection rates have risen again since 1999, together with the rate of patients (children) who were fully vaccinated. In 2002, 85% of Hib cases were in fully vaccinated children. [2] At the very least, it appears, the vaccine quickly wears off and does not confer life-long or even long-term immunity.

Another important consideration is natural immunity vs vaccine induced immunity. 90% of us are believed to carry haemophilus influenzae in us and develop natural immunity through being asymptomatic carriers and through infections from similar organisms. Not only do we acquire lasting immunity against Hib in this way, but also against other organisms through cross-reacting antibodies.

In the UK, Hib vaccination is part of various combined vaccines, such as the 5-in-1 vaccination at 2 months.

References

1. BMJ. Sep 23, 2000; 321(7263): 731–732
2. "Protecting the health of the Nation's children: the benefit of vaccines" – Health Protection Agency

HPV

HPV stands for human papillomavirus, which is sexually transmitted and so common, that anyone who is sexually active will contract the virus at some stage. [2] Usually nothing happens and the immune system simply deals with it. [1,2]

HPV has been linked to cervical cancer through epidemiological studies. It was found that almost all patients with invasive cervical cancer also carry certain types of human papillomavirus, notably types 16 and 18. [8,11] Consequently some researchers now believe that HPV infection is the "first necessary cause" of a human cancer ever identified. In other words, prevent the infection and you prevent cancer. It would be a first and would be exciting if it wasn't for the fact that it has already been disproved. [14]

Cervical cancer constitutes 2% of cancer cases diagnosed in UK women [3] and 1% of cancer deaths, but is the second most common cancer in women worldwide.
The vaccine is meant to protect against the high-risk strains of the virus, thereby preventing the possible development of cervical cancer later on. In the USA the same vaccines are now promoted as protecting against a wide range of other cancers, such as penile and anal cancer.

The NHS website says:

> "Around 970 women died from cervical cancer in 2011 in the UK. It's estimated that about 400 lives could be saved every year in the UK as a result of vaccinating girls before they are infected with HPV." [1]

This is an extremely optimistic outlook. It suggest that almost half of deaths from cervical cancer could be prevented through vaccinations. Time will tell whether this is realistic. Whether it is proportional to vaccinate all young women with the world's riskiest vaccine [7] in order to save an unknown number of lives, possibly none, is up to the reader to decide. In comparison, heart disease killed around 67,000 people in the UK in 2012. [10]

The evidence that HPV vaccination will save any lives is weak.
A study published in 2013 puts it as follows:

> "We carried out a systematic review of HPV vaccine pre- and post-licensure trials to assess the evidence of their effectiveness and safety. We find that HPV vaccine clinical trials design, and data interpretation of both efficacy and safety outcomes, were largely inadequate. Additionally, we note evidence of selective reporting of results from clinical trials (i.e., exclusion of vaccine efficacy figures related to study subgroups in which efficacy might be lower or even negative from peer-reviewed publications). Given this, the widespread optimism regarding HPV vaccines long-term benefits appears to rest on a number of unproven assumptions (or such which are at odd with factual

evidence) and significant misinterpretation of available data. For example, the claim that HPV vaccination will result in approximately 70% reduction of cervical cancers is made despite the fact that the clinical trials data have not demonstrated to date that the vaccines have actually prevented a single case of cervical cancer (let alone cervical cancer death), nor that the current overly optimistic surrogate marker-based extrapolations are justified. Likewise, the notion that HPV vaccines have an impressive safety profile is only supported by highly flawed design of safety trials and is contrary to accumulating evidence from vaccine safety surveillance databases and case reports which continue to link HPV vaccination to serious adverse outcomes (including death and permanent disabilities). We thus conclude that further reduction of cervical cancers might be best achieved by optimizing cervical screening (which carries no such risks) and targeting other factors of the disease rather than by the reliance on vaccines with questionable efficacy and safety profiles." [4]

A (pro-vaccine) study published in 2010 was also realistic and found the vaccine reduced high-grade cervical lesions by 19% during an average follow-up period of 3.6 years, and which hoped that a reduction in cancer rates would follow. [5] We can hope, but it's not a huge reduction and the follow-up period was short compared to the 15-20 years it takes the cancer to develop.

Cancer charity Macmillan is also more cautious on it's website:

"HPV types 16 and 18 are present in about 7 in 10 (70% of) cervical cancers. ... However, as cervical cancer can take many years to develop after HPV infection, it's too early to tell whether the HPV vaccines will help to prevent cervical cancer in the long term." [6]

Meanwhile, almost all infections with high-risk HPV strains pass without causing any symptoms. Only persistent infection with high-risk HPV is linked to cancer. [11]
The only fact which is beyond doubt is that sexual behaviour (or that of partners) is a determining factor and that early first intercourse, multiple partners, etc increase the risk of HPV infection and cervical cancer. [9,13]

Over the last 40 years, cervical cancer mortality has fallen by 75%. The vaccine was only introduced in 2006 but it is to be expected that it will in the future be credited with this fall, as well as any future improvements, should the trend continue. The fact that the drop happened before the vaccine was introduced will be forgotten, just as it was with mortality figures from infectious diseases over the last 100 years.

In summary, cervical cancer is mainly a problem of developing countries and the high-risk HPV strains mainly found in Africa and Asia. [12] In the UK cervical cancer rates are low and the vaccine's protective effects are highly speculative.

The HPV vaccine used in the UK is Gardasil.

References

1. NHS Website January 2014
2. Center for Disease Control and Prevention
3. Cancer Research UK Website January 2014
4. Curr Pharm Des. 2013;19(8):1466-87
5. J Natl Cancer Inst. 2010 Mar 3;102(5):325-39
6. MacMillan Cancer Charity Website January 2014
7. Almost 30,000 adverse events reported to the US VAERS database in only 7 years, constituting 15% of the entire database (MMR has 64,000 reports but spanning more than 25 years).
8. The Journal of Pathology Volume 189, Issue 1, pages 12–19, September 1999
9. Int J Gynecol Cancer. 2012 Nov;22(9):1570-6
10. Office for National Statistics
11. Gynecol Oncol. 2008 Sep;110(3 Suppl 2):S4-7
12. Int J Cancer. 2004 Aug 20;111(2):278-85
13. The epidemiology of human papillomavirus infection and its association with cervical cancer, International Journal of Gynecology and Obstetrics (2006) 94 (Supplement 1), S8–S21
14. J Exp Ther Oncol. 2014;10(4):247-53.

Measles

Measles is a viral infection, usually causing cold-like symptoms, sensitivity to light, fever and a rash. Often neck glands also swell. Measles spreads through sneezes and coughs and is highly infectious.

All symptoms normally resolve without medical intervention after a week or so. Complications are rare and are associated with pre-existing illness, malnutrition and lack of vitamin A.[1] They rarely occur in otherwise healthy and well-nourished children. Once a child has had the disease, it is very unlikely to ever get measles again.

The WHO says:

> "Severe complications from measles can be avoided though supportive care that ensures good nutrition, adequate fluid intake and treatment of dehydration…All children in developing countries diagnosed with measles should receive two doses of vitamin A supplements, given 24 hours apart. This treatment restores low vitamin A levels during measles that occur even in well-nourished children and can help prevent eye damage and blindness. Vitamin A supplements have been shown to reduce the number of deaths from measles by 50%."[1]

During the 2013 outbreak in South Wales, the media portrayed measles as a killer disease and health authorities started a mass-immunisation campaign. Of the 1455[2] total reported cases, only about a third were confirmed to be measles following laboratory tests. [3] Several hundred cases still sounds like a lot but that in itself isn't of concern, as the disease is generally harmless. The media focused on the only death case of the outbreak, a 25 year old male with alcohol problems, who was on a detox and therefore more vulnerable. He appears to have contracted pneumonia as a complication from measles but no one is quite sure if he was even confirmed to have Measles or what the reason of death really was. A BBC article claimed he was advised to take paracetamol against the fever and sent home.[4]
Unfortunately medicating against fever is one of the most common mistakes in treating illness and one which even the NHS website is, at the time of writing, still incorrectly advising. Fever is one of the body's defences against infection and should not be suppressed in most circumstances. Even current (2013) NICE guidelines advice that medications such as paracetamol and ibuprofen should not be given with the sole purpose of reducing fever. [5]

The Health Protection Agency says that 1-6% of measles cases develop pneumonia and about 0.1% encephalitis or blindness. [6] They refer to a WHO document as source [7], which does not itself give any sources. These figures are repeated by a number of official bodies but I have not found any primary source that would confirm their veracity. If they are true, they are very unlikely to include cases of measles which were mild or asymptomatic and which never sought medical attention, as these wouldn't have been reported. Therefore they would represent only 0.1-6% of severe cases and not of the total. They also appear to be referring to a worldwide statistic, including the developing world.

It also has to be remembered that very few of the cases reported as measles are in fact measles. HPA data shows that of all the cases notified as measles, almost none are truly measles when tested. [6]

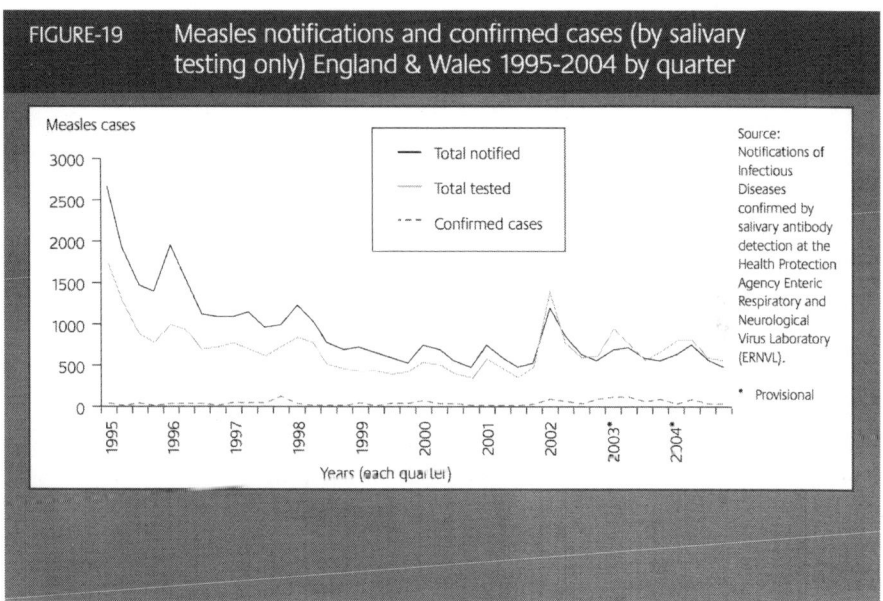

FIGURE-19   Measles notifications and confirmed cases (by salivary testing only) England & Wales 1995-2004 by quarter

Graph from "Protecting the health of the Nation's children: the benefit of vaccines" – Health Protection Agency

Measles ceased to be a killer a long time before the vaccine was introduced and remains so only in developing countries with much lower living conditions than the UK.

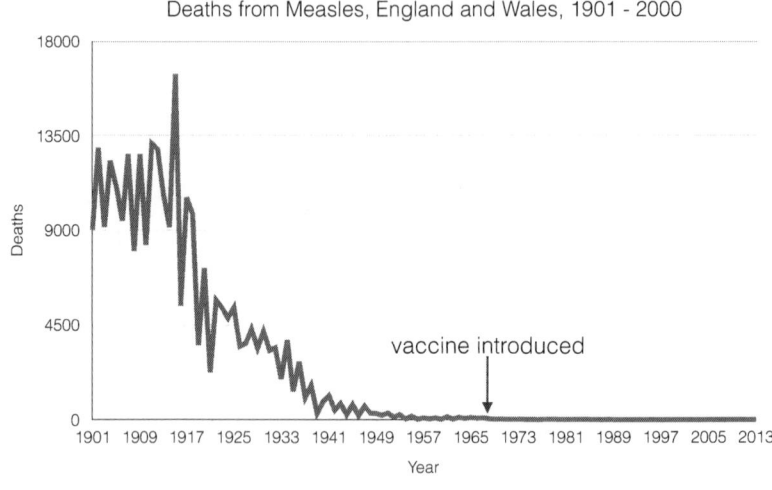

Deaths from Measles, England and Wales, 1901 - 2000

vaccine introduced

Source: Office of National Statistics

In order to convince them of the importance to vaccinate, parents are often shown graphs which only represent part of this data, notably the years after the vaccine was introduced. They are then told that it was the vaccine which caused the reduction in mortality. The following is from an HPA publication [6].

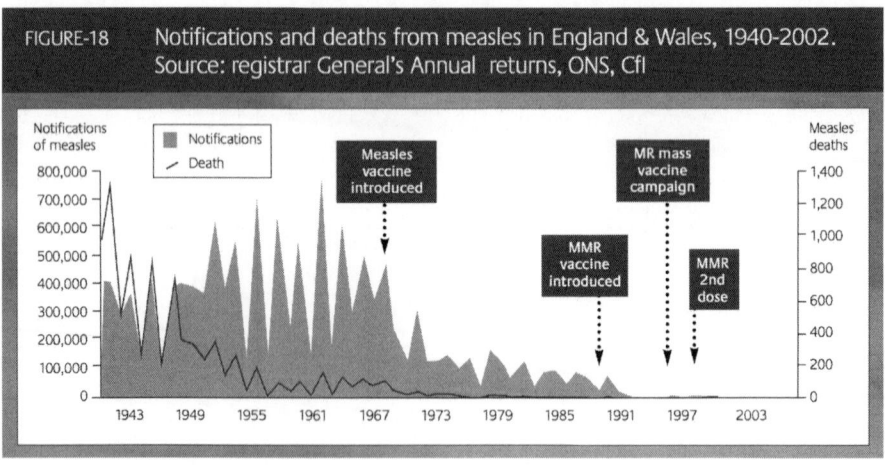

FIGURE-18   Notifications and deaths from measles in England & Wales, 1940-2002. Source: registrar General's Annual returns, ONS, CfI

This graph appears to show a sharp fall in reported cases following the introduction of the vaccine. Whether this was simply the continuation of a century-long trend or whether the vaccine did indeed contribute, remains open to question. Mortality figures are generally more reliable. These, too, took a small dip after the vaccine was introduced but not a remarkable one and as it took 3 years to reach even 50% vaccination coverage, crediting the vaccine with this small improvement is not reliable.

From my research to date, I believe that measles vaccines have shown effectiveness that is remarkably unimpressive. There is data suggesting an 80% rate of effectiveness for a few years but little long-term protection. If we assume that there is indeed a protective effect for a while, this then causes the disease to appear more and more in older age-groups, which will have achieved little. Worryingly, there are many examples of outbreaks in which most of the cases were in fully vaccinated people. A study published in the Archives of Internal Medicine in 1994 "found 18 reports of measles outbreaks in very highly immunized school populations where 71% to 99.8% of students were immunized against measles." The report continues, "Despite these high rates of immunization, 30% to 100% (mean, 77%) of all measles cases in these outbreaks occurred in previously immunized students. In our hypothetical school model, after more than 95% of schoolchildren are immunized against measles, the majority of measles cases occur in appropriately immunized children." [8]

Parents need to be aware of this information when making a vaccination decision and weigh it against the risk from the vaccine.

In the UK, two MMR vaccines are used for the prevention of measles: Priorix and MMRVaxPro.

References

1. World Health Organisation
2. NHS Wales website accessedJanuary 2014
3. Health Protection Agency Website accessedJanuary 2014
4. BBC News Website accessed January 2014
5. National Institute for Health and Care Excellence clinical guidlines CG160
6. Protecting the health of the Nation's children: the benefit of vaccines – Health Protection Agency
7. World Health Organisation. Surveillance guidelines for measles and congenital rubella infection in the WHO European Region. World Health Organisation Regional Office for Europe 2003
8. Arch Intern Med. 1994 Aug 22;154(16):1815-20

Meningitis / Meningococcal Infections

In the UK, the vaccination schedule has recently changed quite a bit regarding Meningococcal vaccinations. The Men C vaccine is a longer established one and used to be referred to (incorrectly) as Meningitis C vaccine, given to infants at 3 months (plus boosters later on). More recently, two more vaccines have been added, one for Men B and one for Men A, C, W, and Y, referred to as Men ACWY vaccine. Men B is a vaccine for infants, while Men ACWY is given in adolescence. [1]

Infections from meningococcal bacteria can cause meningitis and septicaemia. Meningitis is an infection of the protective membranes around the brain and spinal cord and septicaemia is an infection of the blood (blood poisoning).

Most of us carry meningococcus in us at various stages of our lives without becoming ill. This is thought to be important for the development of natural immunity. [2,3,4] Those who do get ill are usually infected by a carrier who did not have any symptoms. It is not known why some get ill from the bacterium (whose proper name is Neisseria meningitidis), so the general state of the immune system must be considered the most important defence.

Men C
The Men C vaccines used in the UK are conjugate vaccines, which were introduced in 1999 because their predecessors did not cause long-term protection or protect young children.

Information published by the Health Protection Agency [5], among others, shows that this hasn't changed for the youngest age group (2-4 months), who are left unprotected after about one year. A booster is therefore given at 12 months.

The HPA estimates the overall short-term vaccine effectiveness at 87% and long-term at 83% for children who were vaccinated as part of a "catch-up campaign" but only 66% effectiveness for children vaccinated as part of the routine programme. Some of this data is based on *estimated* risks of getting ill (comparing vaccinated and unvaccinated groups) and some on antibody response.
The overall routine infant immunisation programme was said to be 66% effective. Confused?

On top of it, the NHS website, at the time of writing, says the vaccine virtually eliminated incidents of disease caused by Men C, a claim often repeated but difficult to reconcile with the low vaccine effectiveness often documented on the same pages. The HPA publication references three studies as sources, none of which were entirely independent of vaccine manufacturers' funding. [5]

The HPA and the study authors acknowledge that meningococcal c related diseases also decreased in unvaccinated children (to the same extent) and in adults who weren't targeted for vaccinations (to a lesser extent). They put it down to the vaccine contributing to herd immunity, thereby protecting also those who were not vaccinated. [5,7]

The Joint Committee on Vaccination and Immunisation reviewed the situation in a 2012 document [6], partly relying on the same researchers. They quote a reduction of 95% in diseases caused by meningococcal C since the vaccine was introduced and carry on summarising various studies, highlighting that the vaccine does not protect infants and young children for long, even with the booster at 12 months. But as there just aren't many cases in this age group, they too conclude that they must be protected by herd immunity.

Despite all this seemingly conflicting information it can't be denied that cases of meningitis from meningococcal infections used to be mainly caused by group C and this has since shifted to group B and to a lesser extend to groups ACWY.

Men B
The new vaccine against Men B infections is Bexsero (see relevant chapter). Considering the reduction in Men C cases, it seems reasonable to expect a similar reduction for Men B. Time will tell but if so, will the burden of disease then not simply shift once again to other groups? In any case the data for Bexsero is far from convincing, which is why the JCVI initially recommended against its introduction. However, some furious lobbying followed and the committee changed its mind. One organisation involved in the lobbying, which happens to be based in my local town, is the charity Meningitis Now. The introduction of the vaccine is to no small part thanks to them and by happy coincidence they receive funding from the manufacturer of Bexsero.

Men ACWY
I have not studied these vaccines in particular.

Disease Risk

There is no doubt that meningococcal infections are bad news. They caused 37 deaths in 2012 and 197 cases of meningitis in 2013 (all age groups). The questions is just whether the vaccine prevents it. The following graph shows mortality figures from 1950 to 2012.

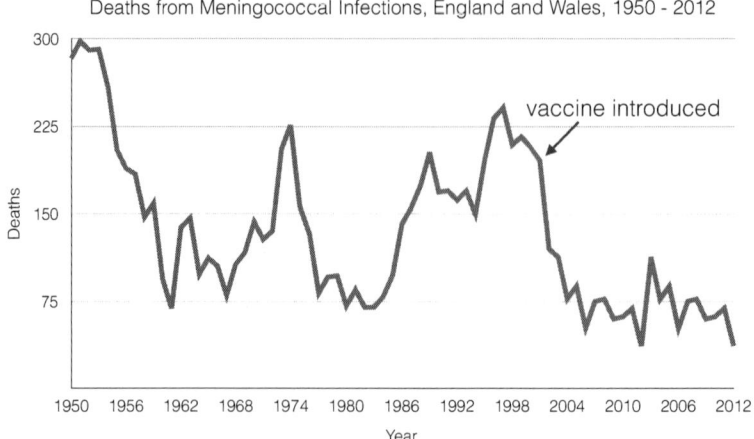

Deaths from Meningococcal Infections, England and Wales, 1950 - 2012

vaccine introduced

Source: Office of National Statistics

We find a big drop following the introduction of the vaccine, though not an unprecedented one.

There are some known risk factors for meningococcal infections and / or meningitis. This is something I have found useful as a parent in order to assess the risk to my children.

Meningitis Risk Factors
• Prematurity / low birth weight increase the risk [8, 9, 10]
• Lack of fever increases the risk [11,12]
• Febrile seizures do **not** pose a significant risk [13]
• In neonates invasive procedures and prior antibiotics use increase the risk [14]
• There is conflicting information whether prior antibiotic use in general increases the risk [15, 16]

I find it noteworthy that patients with "absence of fever have a particularly high risk of an adverse outcome" [11], considering how readily we treat our children with pain medication which also lowers fever. This raises the question to what extend supportive care can reduce the risk to our children in comparison to treatment that suppresses symptoms but does little to address the underlying cause.

Meningococcal Infections Risk Factors
• Preterm birth increases the risk [17, 18]
• Maternal Smoking / passive smoking increase the risk [18, 19, 20, 21, 22, 23, 24, 25, 26]
• Breastfeeding reduces the risk [23, 27]

- Deprivation increases the risk [25, 27, 28]
- Certain lifestyle factors increase the risk. Various studies have identified risk factors often found among students, such as the amount of bar attendance, clubbing, rave attendance, drug taking, etc and correlated them to the risk of adverse outcomes. [17, 21, 29]

Vaccines used in the UK against Meningococcal C infections are Menjugate, NeisVac-C and Meningitec; against Men B infections Bexsero; against Men ACWY infections Nimenrix and Menveo.

References

1. NHS Website accessed January 2014
2. Epidemiol Infect. Jun 2006; 134(3): 556–566
3. J Exp Med. Jun 1, 1969; 129(6): 1327–1348
4. Vaccine. 2001 Jan 8;19(11-12):1327-46
5. Protecting the health of the Nation's children: the benefit of vaccines – Health Protection Agency
6. JCVI statement on the use of meningococcal C vaccines in the routine childhood immunisation programme 29 January 2012
7. BMJ 2003;326:365.1
8. Iran J Child Neurol. 2014 Fall;8(4):46-50.
9. J Infect Dev Ctries. 2013 Feb 15;7(2):73-81
10. Arq Neuropsiquiatr. 2004 Sep;62(3A):630-4
11. J Crit Care. 2014 Jun;29(3):347-50
12. Acta Paediatrica, 91: 391–398
13. Pediatr Emerg Care. 2009 Aug;25(8):494-7
14. Arq Neuropsiquiatr. 2004 Sep;62(3A):630-4
15. Jornal de Pediatria, Volume 89, Issue 3
16. Eur J Clin Microbiol Infect Dis. 2006 Feb;25(2):73-8.
17. BMJ. 2006 Feb 25;332(7539):445-50
18. Int J Epidemiol. 2004 Aug;33(4):816-20.
19. Epidemiol Infect. 1994 Apr; 112(2): 315–328.
20. BMC Public Health. 2012 Dec 10;12:1062
21. Can J Public Health. 2008 Jan-Feb;99(1):46-51.
22. Int J Epidemiol. 2006 Apr;35(2):330-6.
23. Intern Med J. 2004 Aug;34(8):464-8.
24. Epidemiol Infect. 2001 Oct;127(2):261-8.
25. Arch Dis Child. 2000 Aug;83(2):117-21.
26. Pediatr Infect Dis J. 1997 Oct;16(10):979-83.
27. S Afr Med J. 1999 Jan;89(1):56-9.
28. BMC Public Health. 2004 Jul 26;4:30.
29. Pediatr Infect Dis J. 2008 Mar;27(3):193-9

Mumps

Mumps is a mild viral infection similar to a cold. Symptoms can include headaches, fever and the typical swelling of parotid glands, which are located just forward and below the ear. It is spread through coughs and sneezes. Complications are rare. [1] 25-30% of mumps cases are thought to be subclinical, meaning there are no symptoms. [4]

According to Dr Jayne Donegan, a doctor and medical researcher, the British National Formulary stated even just a few years before the MMR vaccine was introduced: "Since mumps and its complications are very rarely serious, there is little indication for the routine use of mumps vaccine". [2]

Complications, rare as they are, can include swollen testicles (orchitis) or ovaries in patients who get mumps after they have gone through puberty. This doesn't cause infertility in females but for males, the NHS says, *out of those who do get orchitis*, "1 in 10 men will experience a drop in their sperm count (the amount of healthy sperm that their body can produce). However, this is very rarely large enough to cause infertility." [3]

Meningitis is often stated as a possible complication and although this is true, this viral meningitis, unlike bacterial meningitis, is much less severe and usually resolves without treatment within 7-10 days, resulting in complete recovery. [18]

In 1980 a Dutch study found that 90% of subjects got mumps before the age of 14. They also found that 25-30% of cases were subclinical (no symptoms). [4] Almost all adults (95%) retained immunity into adulthood.

Today there seems to be a shift into older age groups, where complications are more likely. [5,6,7] This could be a consequence of childhood immunisations shifting the burden of the illness into older patients, in whom the vaccine-induced immunity has waned. This has been seen in other diseases vaccinated against but is, in the case of mumps, difficult to reconcile with the fact that the vaccine does not seem to work in protecting children either.

In fact, mumps vaccination appears to be entirely ineffective.

In Scotland in a 2011 outbreak, 53% of patients were fully vaccinated and another 30% partially so. [7]
In a 2006 nationwide epidemic in the US, 63% of mumps cases happened despite two doses of MMR. [8]
A 2013 study in the US Territory of Guam found that among all the mumps cases in school-age patients, 93% had had 2 doses of MMR.[9]
In Walsall, UK, in 2000, 68% of cases occurred in patients who had had 2 MMR shots and 18.5% in those who had had one dose. [10]
In 1991, an outbreak in Tennessee, USA, occurred in a school where 98% of students were vaccinated. Among 68 students who got ill with mumps, 67 had been vaccinated. The report

concludes: "Most mumps cases were attributable to *primary vaccine failure*."[11]

Another study from the US in 1991 examined mumps cases between 1988 and 1989 during an outbreak in Kansas and found that among primary and secondary school students, 97.6% had been vaccinated.[12]

A 1995 study entitled "Mumps outbreak in a highly vaccinated school population. Evidence for large-scale vaccination failure" found that during an outbreak among a high school population, 95% of the students were vaccinated and out of 54 students who got mumps, 53 were vaccinated. [13]

In a 2007-2008 outbreak among Australian Aboriginals, 52% had had 2 doses of MMR [5] Similar reports from Spain in 2005 [14], Moldova 2008 [6], Spain 2000 [16], USA 2006 [17], Canada [19], among others, all confirm that vaccinating against mumps doesn't work.

Some of the older studies were done when only one dose of MMR was given, and the authors hoped that two doses would work better. But as can be seen from later studies, this was not the case.

Mumps vaccination is part of the MMR vaccine. It seems odd that there is so much controversy over this combined 3-in-1 vaccine when really its use is entirely pointless. It makes no sense to vaccinate against either Mumps or Rubella (Measles is arguable) and the decision whether to give the MMR vaccine should therefore be straight forward.

In the UK, the MMR vaccines in use are: Priorix & MMRVaxPro

References

1. NHS website accessed January 2014
2. Childhood Vaccinatable Diseases And Their Vaccines – A review by Dr Jayne LM Donegan, 2010
3. NHS website accessed January 2014
4. J Hyg (Lond). 1980 December; 85(3): 313–326
5. Med J Aust. 2009 Oct 5;191(7):398-401
6. Pediatr Infect Dis J. 2010 Aug;29(8):703-6
7. Euro Surveill. 2011 Feb 24;16(8)
8. Vaccine. 2009 Oct 19;27(44):6186-95
9. Pediatr Infect Dis J. 2013 Apr;32(4):374-80
10. Int J Infect Dis. 2002 Dec;6(4):283-7
11. J Infect Dis. 1994 Jan;169(1):77-82
12. J Pediatr. 1991 Aug;119(2):187-93
13. Arch Pediatr Adolesc Med 1995 Jul;149(7):774 8
14. Rev Esp Salud Publica. 2007 Nov-Dec;81(6):605-14
15. Pediatr Infect Dis J. 2010 Aug;29(8):703-6
16. Epidemiol Infect. 2002 December; 129(3): 551–556
17. J Med Virol. 2009 Oct;81(10):1819-25
18. Center for Disease Control and Prevention website accessed May 2014
19. CMAJ. 2006 Aug 29;175(5):483-8

Pertussis (Whooping Cough)

Pertussis, or whooping cough, is caused by the bacterium bortadella pertussis. It infects the lungs and airways and causes symptoms which normally start with persistent coughing and which can develop to bouts of coughs that last so long, that when the patient eventually gets to breath in again, a whooping sound can be heard.

Not everyone develops the severe cough and some develop no symptoms at all. Pertussis is spread through the droplets in sneezes and coughs and is very contagious. At worst pertussis can cause pneumonia and death. Babies under the age of 1 are most at risk (3 deaths in 2013).

According to the NHS website, incidents of whooping cough have reduced dramatically since the vaccine was introduced.[1] The figures show that the vaccine may have indeed contributed to the fall, although hardly "dramatically" so, as the number of notifications had been falling for some time. The number of deaths from whooping cough had already fallen by 99% before the vaccine was introduced.

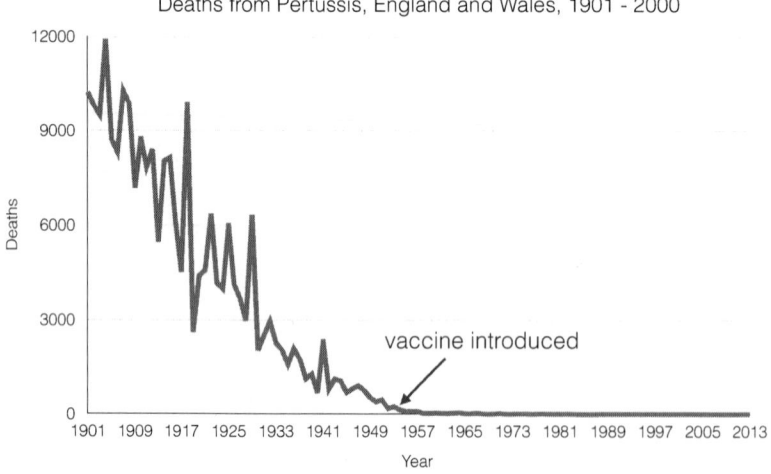

Deaths from Pertussis, England and Wales, 1901 - 2000

Source: Office of National Statistics

When considering whether to vaccinate, it is important to note that getting whooping cough naturally, really does make the patient immune to the disease for the rest of their lives. The vaccine does not, and has been struggling with "waning immunity" and low effectiveness (ranging from 13% – 85% effectiveness) [2,3,10,11,12]. This is thought to be due to the body producing a type of antibody called Immunoglobulin A (IgA) only when pertussis is naturally contracted. This means that if the vaccine is used, boosters are required to "refresh" the "immunity". The more research is being done, the more it is becoming clear that unless we keep vaccinating against pertussis for the rest of a person's life, immunity will wear off and whooping cough will instead re-emerge in older age groups – a trend already evident. [4,5,7,11,12]

Outbreaks of whooping cough keep happening all over the world in a fairly regular cycle of 44 months, which the bacterium seems to be cycling through. When it becomes virulent, outbreaks happen even in highly vaccinated populations.[6,7,13,14,16]

A 2014 study from Canada found that of the suspected pertussis cases that actually were confirmed to be pertussis (which was only an average of 7% of reported cases) 81% had an immunisation record and of those, half were fully immunised.[6]
In another study in Wisconsin, 84% of patients had received 5 or more (!) doses of pertussis vaccine but still got ill.[7]
Longer ago in Shetland in the 1970s it was found that vaccinated children were as likely to get ill as unvaccinated ones. [13]
The same was found in Oklahoma in the 1980s. [15]
And during a 1992 pertussis outbreak in Massachusetts, 96% of students had received four or more doses of pertussis-containing vaccine. [16]
Even an official CDC survey of pertussis cases in 2013 showed that most patients were vaccinated. [22]

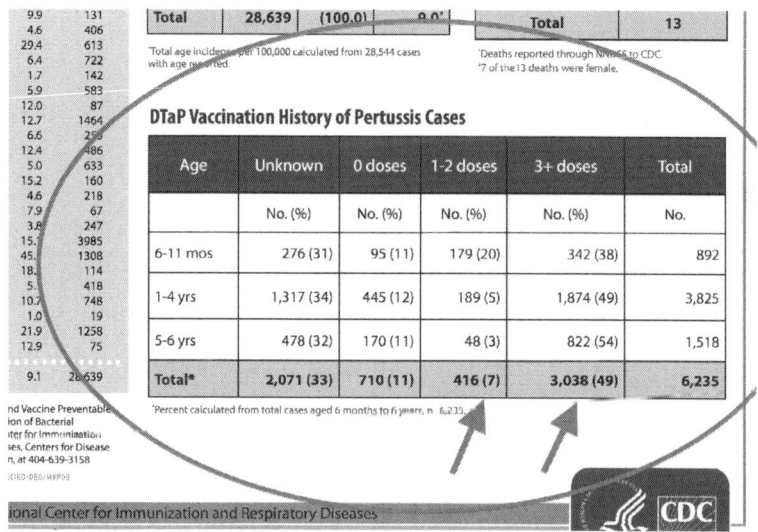

DTaP Vaccination History of Pertussis Cases

Age	Unknown	0 doses	1-2 doses	3+ doses	Total
	No. (%)	No. (%)	No. (%)	No. (%)	No.
6-11 mos	276 (31)	95 (11)	179 (20)	342 (38)	892
1-4 yrs	1,317 (34)	445 (12)	189 (5)	1,874 (49)	3,825
5-6 yrs	478 (32)	170 (11)	48 (3)	822 (54)	1,518
Total*	2,071 (33)	710 (11)	416 (7)	3,038 (49)	6,235

*Percent calculated from total cases aged 6 months to 6 years, n=6,235.

The acellular pertussis vaccine is so useless that reintroduction of the notorious whole-cell vaccine is now being considered in some countries.[8] The whole-cell pertussis component of the old DTP vaccine caused so many severe side-effects, that it was eventually replaced by the current vaccine, which is believed to be safer.

In addition to worries regarding permanent neurological damage, studies were finding links to asthma and allergies later on in life [17,18,19], although other studies found no link [20,21] (data was significantly "adjusted" by the study authors of [21]).

The Health Protection Agency puts it in a way that can only be called highly diplomatic, when it says that DTP was "a very effective vaccine but is associated with a relatively high level of non-serious reactions...Whilst these children suffered no long-term problems there was motivation to find an alternative vaccine that was just as effective but less likely to lead to reactions."[9]

But considering that many of the above quoted studies precede the change from the whole cell to the acellular vaccine, it is clear that neither version is effective.

Vaccines used in the UK against Whooping Cough are Pediacel, Infanrix-IPV and Repevax.

References

1. NHS Website accessed January 2014
2. Trends Microbiol. 2014 Feb;22(2):49-52
3. Cochrane Database Syst Rev. 2011 Jan 19;(1):CD001478
4. Am J Prev Med. 2007 Mar;32(3):177-185
5. J Am Board Fam Med. 2006 Nov-Dec;19(6):603-11
6. BMC Infect Dis. 2014 Jan 30;14(1):48
7. Arch Pediatr Adolesc Med. 2008 Jan;162(1):79-85
8. Indian Pediatr. 2013 Nov 8;50(11):1001-9
9. Protecting the health of the Nation's children: the benefit of vaccines – Health Protection Agency
10. Vaccine. 2012 Jan 11;30(3):544-51
11. Clin Infect Dis. 2012 Jun;54(12):1730-5
12. Pediatrics. 2006 Sep;118(3):978-84
13. Br Med J. 1979 June 16; 1(6178): 1601–1603
14. Br Med J (Clin Res Ed). 1984 January 21; 288(6412): 232–233
15. CDC MMWR January 13, 1984
16. CDC MMWR March 26, 1993
17. J Manipulative Physiol Ther. 2000 Feb;23(2):81-90
18. Epidem 1997; 8: 678-680
19. Primal Health Research Newsletter 1997; 4(4): 3-6
20. Vaccine. 2006 Mar 15;24(12):2035-42. Epub 2005 Nov 28
21. BMJ. 2004 Apr 17;328(7445):925-6. Epub 2004 Mar 19
22. 2013 Final Pertussis Surveillance Report - CDC

Pneumococcal diseases

Pneumococcal diseases are caused by the bacterium Streptococcus pneumoniae, of which there are more than 90 different kinds, called serotypes. These can cause a wide variety of infections, not just pneumonia, including meningitis, blood poisoning, otitis media and many others.

Streptococcus pneumoniae is normally present in our bodies without causing any problems but it can become virulent given the right circumstances.
Mild forms of pneumococcal infections do not require medical attention. Severe forms currently respond very well to antibiotics, although an increase in antibiotics resistance is being noticed. The risk is low but there is a risk. In 2012, 6 infants died from infections of this kind and every year the bacterium causes around 60 cases of meningitis in all age groups.

The vaccine efficacy is generally between 0% and 40%, depending on the information source, the exact age-group and the exact outcome measure, with the occasional 70%-80% peak results. [1,2,3] Vaccines appear to work fairly well for the right serotypes, those contained in the vaccine, but there is little effect on non-vaccines serotypes.

A Canadian study published in 2010 also looked at occurrence of "complicated pneumonia in children" and found a slight increase since the introduction of the vaccine, i.e. the situation got slightly worse.[4]

Another study, looking at the overall incidents of invasive pulmonary diseases in the same area, found the vaccine effective for the serotypes it contained. But for other serotypes, incidents increased. [5]

Many studies have shown this shift, i.e. the serotypes against which we vaccinate are less often the cause for illness and patients instead get ill from non-vaccine serotypes. [4,5,6,7,8] Due to this, some researchers are hoping to be able to produce future vaccines that protect against all types. [9]

The following shows the number of reported *cases* of Pneumococcal Meningitis.

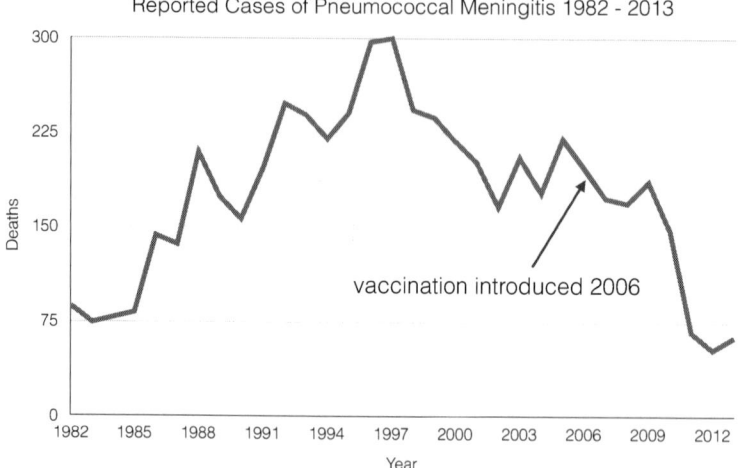

Reported Cases of Pneumococcal Meningitis 1982 - 2013

vaccination introduced 2006

Source: Office of National Statistics

It is not known what causes the streptococcus pneumonia bacterium to become a pathogen when it otherwise lives harmlessly inside us. It is therefore reasonable to assume, in the absence of evidence to the contrary, that general health and the overall state of our immune system are crucial.

The vaccine currently used in the UK is Prevnar 13, which aims at 13 of over 90 serotypes of this bacterium.

References

1. Pediatr Infect Dis J. 2009 Jun;28(6):455-62
2. Lancet. 2005 Mar 26-Apr 1;365(9465):1139-46
3. Emerg Infect Dis. 2013 Apr;19(4):589-97
4. Eur J Pediatr. 2010 Sep;169(9):1123-8
5. Clin Infect Dis. 2009 Jul 15;49(2):205-12
6. Clin Microbiol Infect. 2009 Nov;15(11):1013-9
7. Pediatr Infect Dis J. 2013 Feb;32(2):e45-53
8. Pediatr Infect Dis J. 2012 Mar;31(3):249-54
9. Cell Mol Life Sci. 2013 Sep;70(18):3303-26

Polio

Poliomyelitis is caused by infection with poliovirus, which is usually spread from person to person, particularly in conditions of poor hygiene. Fewer than 0.1% of those infected as children actually suffer paralysis.

The NHS describes polio as a disease of the past and says that the last case of natural infection in the UK happened in 1984. The few cases since then where either brought in from other countries or caused by the live oral vaccine. [1] (HPA data shows no cases acquired overseas between 1994 and 2003, so all were acquired from the vaccine in this time period. [2])

Since 2004 the UK uses the inactivated polio vaccine. This is just as well, as there have been plenty of documented cases internationally, where polio outbreaks occurred immediately after mass-vaccination campaigns with the live vaccine (see for example [3]), leading researchers to wonder why these had happened despite the vaccinations but logically they must have happened because of them. The 1988 Oman outbreak is often cited, where most children had received at least 3 doses of the vaccine and where areas with high vaccination coverage had the highest attack rate and vice versa. [3] A similar vaccine-caused outbreak didn't happen here in the UK. Better living conditions are a reasonable explanation.

The inactivated version now in use cannot cause the disease.

Unlike other diseases, polio did not go through a long decline before vaccinations started. Polio was only recognised as a separate disease in England in 1911 and saw a huge increase in the 1940s-1960s before disappearing again. Vaccines were introduced in 1956 and 1962.

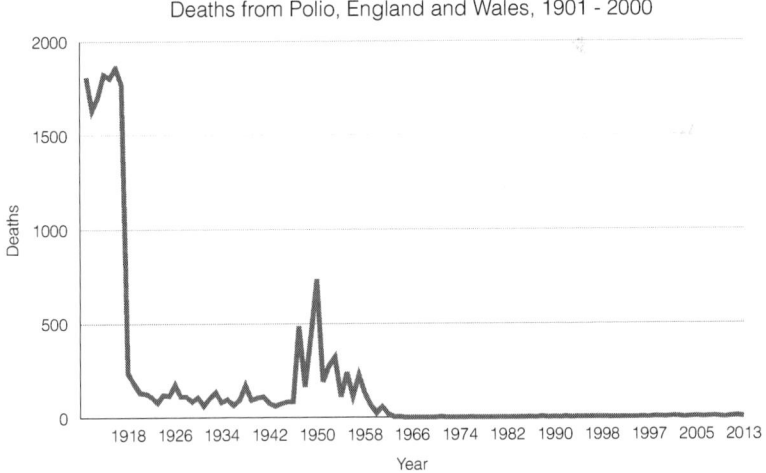

Deaths from Polio, England and Wales, 1901 - 2000

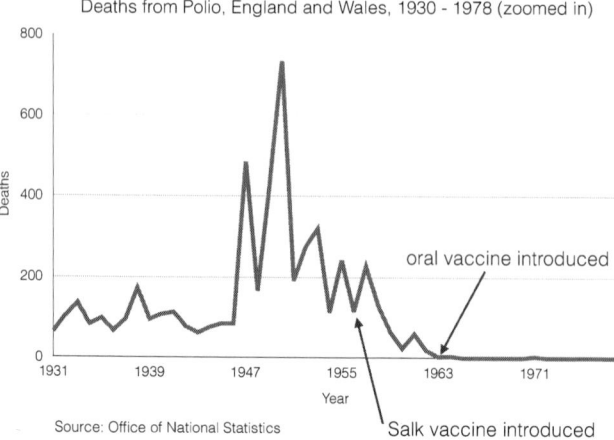

Deaths from Polio, England and Wales, 1930 - 1978 (zoomed in)

oral vaccine introduced

Source: Office of National Statistics

Salk vaccine introduced

Why the disease spiked in the 1940s and 1950s is not known. A fact also not widely known is that the diagnostic parameters for Polio were radically changed at the time the vaccine was first introduced in the US. This re-definition alone caused most Polio cases to be removed from the statistics and the vaccine was credited with the improvement.[5]

Parents making their vaccination decision should consider the almost non-existent risk from polio in the UK. Vaccines used in the UK against Polio are: Pediacel, Infanrix-IPV, Repevax and Revaxis.

Meanwhile the live oral vaccine is being used for large-scale vaccination campaigns in countries like India, where cases of polio are said to have dramatically fallen, while authorities record an equally dramatic *rise* in acute flaccid paralysis [4], meaning people are still getting paralysed, but apparently not from polio.

References
1. NHS website accessed March 2014
2. Protecting the health of the Nation's children: the benefit of vaccines – Health Protection Agency
3. Lancet. 1991 Sep 21;338(8769):715-20
4. The Times of India website accessed May 2014
5. The Present Status of Polio Vaccines, Illinois Medical Journal, August 1960

Rotavirus infections

Rotavirus can cause gastroenteritis, commonly known as a "vomiting bug". The NHS says rotavirus is a "common" cause for gastroenteritis and that although "most children recover at home within a few days", about 2% end up in hospital for dehydration. [1] Rotavirus has also been blamed for hundreds of thousands of infant deaths world wide and 20-60 deaths a year in the USA before the vaccine was introduced. [2] Rotavirus can also be asymptomatic.

The fact that diarrhoea is a leading cause of infant deaths in developing countries is no secret.

Gastroenteritis can be caused by many organisms other than rotavirus and although official sources say rotavirus is the leading cause, how do they know? Doctors don't generally test for it when a child comes in with diarrhoea, even in the developed world, let alone the countries where infant diarrhoea is a killer.

In a study published in 2011, only 13.8% of children admitted to Jos university teaching hospital in Nigeria with acute diarrhoea were found to be infected with rotavirus. [3]
A study published in 2004 examining children hospitalised in Poland for acute diarrhoea found that 16.1% were infected with rotavirus.[4]
In Tunis during 2007, 25% of acute gastroenteritis were due to rotavirus. [5]

However other studies have found higher rates,
A French study published in 2000 found 37.1% of infants hospitalised for gastroenteritis had rotavirus in their stool. [6]
A Polish study came to a rate of 29.6% [7] and a multi-centre study covering Austria, Germany and Switzerland came to 27-37%. [10]

All these studies were done in hospitals, showing that rotavirus is a problem in hospitals. Indeed rotavirus infections are often acquired in hospital (so called nosocomial rotavirus infections). Another French study published in 2007 found 13.9% of rotavirus infections were acquired in hospital. [8]
Authors of a Spanish study claimed "Between 20% and 50% of gastroenteritis cases caused by rotavirus and astrovirus are of nosocomial origin.", i.e. hospital-acquired [9] and the above mentioned study covering Austria, Germany and Switzerland found that when gastroenteritis was acquired in hospital, 49% – 69% were caused by rotavirus.

What about outside of hospital?

A study published in 2013 examined 710 patients with diarrhoea in displaced communities in Sudan and found 12% were due to rotavirus. [11]
In Nigeria researchers conducted house-to-house visits and found rotavirus in 9% of people suffering from diarrhoea. [12]

This data suggests that even in developing countries, rotavirus is only responsible for a small part of diarrhoea cases.

Almost everyone gets infected by rotavirus by the age of 5 and although we do not necessarily get immune after the first time, we do acquire natural immunity gradually and not just for one but for multiple serotypes of the virus. [13,14] Infants often show no symptoms at all [14]. In the UK, it is rare that children with gastroenteritis need medical care and as treatment only consists of keeping the patient hydrated, this can usually be done at home and the child will usually recover within a few days. Breastfeeding has a beneficial effect but does not provide complete protection. [14] Considering the risk of contracting the virus in hospital, it may well be that if a child is admitted with non-rotavirus gastroenteritis, it will get the virus while in hospital.

Children do die from Rotavirus in the UK but the average mortality is less than one per year.

This information may help parents decide whether to see rotavirus as one of many "tummy bugs" or a serious threat to their children's health. The vaccine does not provide 100% protection but there is data showing that it does work. Studies have variously found 70% [15], 82% [16] and 91%[17] vaccine effectiveness. One study even found that one vaccine had reduced hospital admissions for acute rotavirus gastroenteritis by 100%, an amazing result, which may partially be due to the fact that the researchers were on the manufacturer's payroll. [18]

In the UK, the vaccine used to prevent rotavirus infections is Rotarix..

References
1. NHS website accessed May 2014
2. CDC Website accessed March 2014C
3. Virol J. 2011; 8: 233
4. Przegl Epidemiol. 2004;58(3):475-81
5. Tunis Med. 2009 Sep;87(9):599-602
6. Arch Pediatr. 2000 Oct;7(10):1050-8
7. Przegl Epidemiol. 2008;62(3):557-63
8. Med Mal Infect. 2007 Jan;37(1):61-6. Epub 2006 Dec 5
9. An Pediatr (Barc). 2004 Apr;60(4):337-43
10. Pediatr Infect Dis J. 2001 Aug;20(8):784-91
11. BMC Infect Dis. 2013 May 8;13:209
12. Ann Afr Med. 2008 Dec;7(4):168-74
13. Pediatr Infect Dis J. 2009 Mar;28(3 Suppl):S54-6
14. J Med Microbiol. 1995 Dec;43(6):397-404
15. Clin Infect Dis. 2013 Jul;57(1):13-20
16. J Pediatr. 1985 Aug;107(2):189-94
17. Pediatrics. 2013 Jul;132(1):e25-33
18. Pediatrics. 2010 Feb;125(2):e208-13

Rubella

Rubella is a mild viral infection which most children used to get as a childhood illness. It is also known as German measles and symptoms are normally similar to a cold, including fever. A rash can also develop, which normally lasts for 24 hrs to a few days. [1] A person who has had Rubella usually acquires life-long immunity.

The only time when Rubella becomes a problem is when women contract it during early pregnancy. However, vaccinations are done in infancy and often no longer protect women by the time they are of childbearing age.[2,3,6]

Rubella can affect the fetal development when the mother gets the disease in the first or sometimes second trimester of pregnancy, which can then result in birth defects, so-called congenital rubella syndrome or CRS.

The Health Protection Agency, the the British Paediatric Surveillance Unit and other sources say that there were 200 – 300 cases of congenital rubella per year before the vaccine came in and that this number has since dramatically fallen, so that there are now very few cases. [4,5] Proper surveillance of congenital rubella syndrome only started after the vaccine was introduced and I have not been able to find a primary source for the quoted number of 200-300. Without a source, it is impossible to check if the statement is true. Official statistics for the time period following the introduction of the vaccine do suggest a gradual decline, which could be due to vaccinations.

But information from the CDC [6] points to the increasing number of rubella cases in older age groups:

> "Until recently, there was no predominant age group for rubella cases. From 1982 through 1992, approximately 30% of cases occurred in each of three age groups: younger than 5, 5–14, and 15–39 years. Adults 40 years of age and older typically accounted for less than 10% of cases. However, since 1993, persons 15–39 years of age have accounted for more than half the cases. In 2003, this age group accounted for 71% of all reported cases."

This means that more and more rubella cases occur at an age when women could become pregnant. This is difficult to reconcile with the claim that the vaccine has reduced the cases of CRS. In fact, a Canadian study published in December 2014 found that Rubella vaccinations increased the risk of CRS due to their negative impact on natural immunity.[8]

When researchers looked into a rubella outbreak in Brazil in 2000, they found that "The incidence among persons aged 12 to 19 years was increased 3.7-fold relative to children aged 1 to 4 years." [2] They concluded: "Vaccination among school age children was insufficient to prevent a rubella outbreak among young adults that resulted in the occurrence of at least 5 cases of CRS", which confirms that vaccinating in infancy and early childhood simply does not reduce the risk of CRS.

In all the studies I found concerning rubella outbreaks, only a small fraction of reported/suspected cases of rubella and or CRS actually turned out to be so when laboratory tests were conducted.

There is no reason why the rubella vaccine should be given in infancy and early childhood, nor is there any reason why children should not contract the disease naturally. Doing so would be a much more reliable and side-effect free prevention of rubella in later life. Including the vaccine in the childhood vaccination programme is logistically convenient, especially as it is included in the MMR combined vaccine, but does not otherwise make sense. In order to prevent CRS, girls could be examined for rubella antibodies in their early teens and vaccination considered then. They may not need it and if they do, a single dose of rubella vaccine is supposed to be enough in 95% of cases according to the WHO [7], avoiding the need for multiple MMR doses.

In the UK, two MMR vaccines are used for the prevention of Rubella: Priorix and MMRVaxPro.

References
1. NHS website accessed April 2014
2. Pediatr Infect Dis J. 2003 Apr;22(4):323-9
3. J Pediatr (Rio J). 2007 Sep-Oct;83(5):415-21
4. Protecting the health of the Nation's children: the benefit of vaccines – Health Protection Agency
5. BMJ 1999;318:769
6. CDC website accessed May 2014
7. WHO Fact sheet N°367, July 2012
8. Vaccine. 2014 Dec 19. pii: S0264-410X(14)01651-X

Tetanus

Tetanus is another bacterial infection, this time caused by toxins produced by the bacterium Clostridium tetani. Infections are rare in the UK but complications can be serious and even fatal.

The bacterium causing tetanus is very resilient and can live in the environment for many years. However, it only produces toxins in anaerobic conditions, which is why it is associated with deep wounds which cannot easily be reached by oxygen.
Symptoms can include muscle spasms and stiffness (including in the jaw muscles – lockjaw), difficulty swallowing and fever. Symptoms can be limited to the injury site and not develop further. They can also be much more serious and lead to a quick death.

Tetanus mortality, like that of other diseases, had already reduced by 90-100% in the UK and US by the time the vaccine was introduced and/or put into wider use. This was likely due to improvements in wound hygiene as well as other treatments. This suggests that the low risk of contracting tetanus would still be very low even if there was no vaccination. There is still very high mortality for infants contracting tetanus in the developing world but this is due to hygiene issues at birth.[2]

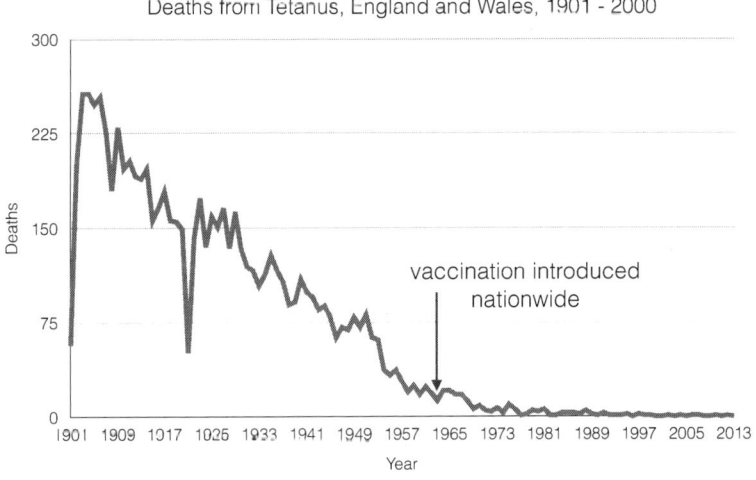

Deaths from Tetanus, England and Wales, 1901 - 2000

Source: Office of National Statistics

Is the vaccine effective?

In one 1993 study, 4 out of 5 children with tetanus were described as adequately vaccinated.[3] These 5 children, as well as 101 adults, were the only ones to get the disease in Finland over a 16 year period. The paper describes the symptoms as mild and implies this may have been due to the vaccinations, compared to the often unvaccinated population in the developing world. But this is a highly speculative statement, as the difference in hygiene and other living conditions is much more likely to be the reason.

US data for all cases of tetanus between 1995 – 1997 shows that 24.8% of patients had had at least one dose of tetanus vaccine but only 12.4% had 3 or more doses. 21.5% were unvaccinated and of 53.7% the vaccination status was not known. [4] The authors highlight the fact that of all the cases only 13% were in fully vaccinated patients but the fact that as many again had been partially vaccinated and that of more than half, they simply didn't know if they were vaccinated or not, was left to a table in the appendix. It is noted that 4 out of 14 deaths occurred in the "known unvaccinated" and only 1 in the "known vaccinated". 9 deaths were among those of unknown vaccination status.

In 1992 a publication in *Neurology* stated

> Severe (grade III) tetanus occurred in three immunized patients who had high serum levels of anti-tetanus antibody. The disease was fatal in one patient. One patient had been hyperimmunized to produce commercial tetanus immune globulin. Two patients had received immunizations 1 year before presentation.[8]

Most official sources claim that the tetanus vaccine is highly effective, based, on looking for an antibody response to the vaccine and then assuming that this means the patient is now immune. But the above cases show that such an assumption is unfounded.

One thing is at least undisputed: Tetanus is a disease of the older age-groups and not primarily one that affects children [4,5,6], excluding obviously neonatal tetanus in developing countries, which is a hygiene issue and not one that affects developed countries.
On average there are 5 cases of (not deaths from) Tetanus in the UK per year and fewer than 1 mortality per year on average. The last time a *child* died from Tetanus in the UK was in 1973.

To summarise, we can say that there is conflicting data over the effectiveness of the vaccine. We know that tetanus can be a very serious condition and that hygiene and wound care are by far the most important factor in reducing risk. We also know that mainly adults are affected. This could be due to the vaccine initially being effective and then wearing off, in which case we are left with a choice between life-long boosters or relying on natural immunity.

Does natural immunity to tetanus exist?
We know that the vaccine causes the body to produce antibodies against the tetanus toxin and

that despite this, one can still get ill from tetanus. We also know that tetanus toxin antibodies occur naturally in unvaccinated individuals. A thorough study in 1985 found antibodies to tetanus toxin in 98% of unvaccinated individuals [7] but that too, of course, doesn't equate to immunity. Antibodies alone never have explained much on their own. The risk from tetanus remains strongly linked to the overall circumstances, such as wound hygiene and overall health and the state of the immune system in general.

Tetanus vaccination in the UK is part of the 5 in 1 Pediacel vaccine and other booster combinations. When making a vaccination decision, the risk-benefit analysis has to include the risks from these combined vaccines.

References
1. NHS website accessed February 2014
2. UNICEF website accessed May 2014
3. Dev Med Child Neurol. 1993 Apr;35(4):351-5
4. MMWR CDC Surveill Summ. 1998 Jul 3;47(2):1-13
5. Przegl Epidemiol. 2013;67(2):253-4, 357-8
6. Changgeng Yi Xue Za Zhi. 1990 Dec;13(4):296-303
7. Infect Immun. 1985 April; 48(1): 267–268
8. Neurology. 1992 Apr;42(4):761-4

Vaccines

Bexsero

Generic Name: Meningococcal group B Vaccine (rDNA, component, adsorbed)
Manufacturer: Novartis

Bexsero Vaccine Safety

The product information published on the website of the European Medicines Agency says 14 safety studies exist, involving 8776 individuals including 5849 under the age of 2. [3]
The document is short on detail but the US version of the Bexsero product information says Novartis conducted four safety trials involving a total of 3058 individuals. In only one of these a saline placebo was used as control for the first dose of Bexsero. For the second dose the control was another vaccine. In the other trials the "placebo" groups received aluminium hydroxide and other vaccines instead of a true placebo. The published prescribing information lists "solicited" (pre-determined) adverse reactions for the one trial where a saline placebo was used. In almost all cases Bexsero recipients suffered a much higher rate of side-effects, especially for sever reactions, compared to placebo.

Severe Pain: Bexsero 20 - Placebo 2
Severe Fatigue: Bexsero 4 - Placebo 0
Severe Nausea: Bexsero 4 - Placebo 0
Severe Myalgia: Bexsero 12 - Placebo 1
Severe Athralgia: Bexsero 2 - Placebo 0
Severe Headache Bexsero 4 - Placebo 1

Unsolicited Serious Adverse Events were apparently reported by 0.8% of vaccine recipients but no further details was given. [2]

None of these four trials involved infants. However, an infants trial was conducted later on by the *European MenB Vaccine Study Group* on behalf of and with funding from Novartis. Groups of infants were either given MenB vaccine plus a range of routine childhood vaccinations, or only routine vaccinations. Out of 1885 infants, serious adverse events were reported in 158 but only 20 were thought to be possibly vaccine related by the study investigators. There were two cases of Kawasaki disease. [5]

The European Medicines Agency admits in its assessment that there is "insufficient knowledge about immunological and/or autoimmune reactions" and that "data in elderly or immunosuppressed individuals is missing." [1] Assessing the safety of the vaccine was left to the post-marketing experience. In other words, we will find out once Bexsero has been injected into large numbers of infants as part of the routine childhood immunisation programme.

The UK's JCVI called the data "too limited to identify rare reactions to the vaccine." [4]

Bexsero Vaccine Efficacy

Bexsero was tested for immunogenicity (antibody response) only. No efficacy data is available and this was left to the post-marketing period. Antibody counts decline rapidly in infants [4] and no proof of protective levels was provided for more than 6 months following the last dose, according to the European Medicines Agency.

Contraindications according to the manufacturer

"Hypersensitivity, including severe allergic reaction, to any component of the vaccine, or after a previous dose of BEXSERO."
Also listed are precautions applicable to the administration of vaccines in general.

Adverse reactions according to the manufacturer
(for infants and children)

Metabolism and nutrition disorders
Very common: eating disorders

Immune system disorders
Not known: allergic reactions (including anaphylactic reactions)

Nervous system disorders
Very common: sleepiness, unusual crying
Uncommon: seizures (including febrile seizures)

Vascular disorders
Uncommon: pallor (rare after booster)
Rare: Kawasaki syndrome

Gastrointestinal disorders
Very common: diarrhoea, vomiting (uncommon after booster)

Skin and subcutaneous tissue disorders
Very common: rash (children aged 12 to 23 months) (uncommon after booster)
Common: rash (infants and children 2 to 10 years of age)
Uncommon: eczema
Rare: urticaria

General disorders and administration site conditions
Very common: fever ($\geq 38°C$), injection site tenderness (including severe injection site tenderness defined as crying when injected limb is moved), injection site erythema, injection site swelling, injection site induration, irritability

Uncommon: fever (≥40°C)
Not known: blisters at or around the injection site

Ingredients

Recombinant Neisseria meningitidis group B NHBA/NadA/fHbp proteins
Outer membrane vesicles (OMV) from Neisseria meningitidis group B
strain NZ98/254
Aluminium hydroxide
Sodium chloride Histidine
Sucrose
Water for injections

References
1. European Medicines Agency Assessment Report
2. Bexsero Prescribing Information
3. Summary of product characteristics, European Medicines Agency
4. Bexsero interim statement, Joint Committee on Vaccinations and Immunisations
5. Gossger et. al. JAMA. 2012;307(6):573-582

Fluenz Tetra

Manufacturer: MedImmune/AstraZeneca
Generic name: Influenza vaccine (live attenuated, nasal)

Fluenz Tetra Safety

The European Medicines Agency considers the safety profile of Fluenz Tetra as similar to Fluenz, its predecessor. It says it did not know whether repeat use of the vaccine may cause allergic reactions, nor whether the rate of serious side-effects can be adequately measured with the proposed post-authorisation safety studies. But they conclude: "However the ten years long marketing experience in the US has not raised major concerns for the time being."

The EMA previously evaluated safety trials for Fluenz and considered it safe.
A study published in 2008 looked at increased risk to children "with history of intermittent wheezing" and found no increased risk from the vaccines. [1] Other studies similarly looked into vaccines and the risk from acute respiratory illness and found no link. [2]

Conversely, a large study published in 2004 found: "For reactive airway disease a significant increased relative risk was observed in children 18 to 35 months of age… The individual diagnostic categories of upper respiratory infection, musculoskeletal pain, otitis media with effusion and adenitis/adenopathy had at least one analysis that achieved a significant increased risk ratio". [4] Children are also almost twice as likely to suffer gastrointestinal symptoms after vaccination as the placebo group, mainly after the first dose, but much less so after subsequent doses. [3]

These examples are typical for the data available, which varies widely from publication to publication and often arriving at opposing results.

The US Vaccines Adverse Events Reporting System (VAERS) currently contains 5500 events for this type of vaccine from this manufacturer. About a fifth were classified as serious. Worst case, if all the reports were confirmed and assuming an under-reporting ratio of 5 in 100, this would make around 20,000 serious adverse events out of millions of doses administered.

However, it should also be noted that in recent years, flu vaccinations made up 58% of all cases where compensation was paid under the US National Vaccine Injury Compensation Program.[7]

Inactivated flu vaccines are said to be unable to cause flu, however, very common side-effects are very much flu-like. Up to 1 in 10 recipients will suffer fever and muscle aches and between 1 in 10 and everyone will suffer a runny or stuffy nose, reduced appetite, weakness and headaches. [5] The benefit of avoiding flu vs getting flu-like side-effects plus the risk of other side-effects has to be questioned. As this vaccine is a live vaccine, vaccinated children can infect others with the "weakened" viruses contained in Fluenz Tetra.

Fluenz Tetra Efficacy

The European Medicines Agency says the manufacturer showed them data proving that Fluenz Tetra compared well to Fluenz, which they see as having an established effectiveness. This is called a non-inferiority study. They also say data was presented proving that trial subjects developed antibodies to the strains in the vaccine.

However it should be born in mind that antibody response (immunogenicity) is only assumed to constitute immunity and that it has repeatedly been shown that this is a flawed assumption, as people with high antibody counts can and do get ill. The regulator acknowledges this to some extend, saying there remain uncertainties. They also point out that although Fluenz Tetra caused an antibody response similar to that of Fluenz, this was lower than expected and not much higher than baseline values. The EMA concludes: "The efficacy of the vaccine following repeated yearly revaccinations would benefit from further evidence.
Overall these uncertainties are expected to be addressed in the post-authorisation effectiveness study described in the RMP."

Manufacturer MedImmune says it conducted 9 efficacy trials for Fluenz, involving over 20,000 children and that in 3 studies Fluenz proved to be better than other, injectable vaccines. In the 9 studies overall they recorded efficacy of between 46% and 100% depending on age group and whether the flu virus strain in circulation was similar to the strain of the vaccine.

The European Medicines Agency says: "The studies in adults showed that Fluenz may have some benefits compared with placebo but the results were inconsistent. Some studies also suggested that Fluenz was not as effective as the comparator inactivated vaccine in adults." [6] But they accept the above figures for children.
I cannot comment much on these studies, as the manufacturer conducted them and remained in full control of the data. They must be viewed with some caution, due to the manufacturer's self-interest. I have instead conducted my own review on the effectiveness of vaccinating with live attenuated influenza vaccines, which can be found in the chapter on flu.

Contraindications (according to the package insert/patient information leaflet)

• Hypersensitivity to the active substances or to any of the excipients listed in section 6.1 (e.g. gelatin), or to gentamicin (a possible trace residue), to eggs or to egg proteins (e.g. ovalbumin).

• Children and adolescents with clinical immunodeficiency due to conditions or immunosuppressive therapy such as: acute and chronic leukaemias; lymphoma; symptomatic HIV infection; cellular immune deficiencies; and high-dose corticosteroids. Fluenz Tetra is not contraindicated for use in individuals with asymptomatic HIV infection; or individuals who are receiving topical/inhaled corticosteroids or low-dose systemic corticosteroids or those receiving corticosteroids as replacement therapy, e.g. for adrenal insufficiency.

- Children and adolescents younger than 18 years of age receiving salicylate therapy because of the association of Reye's syndrome with salicylates and wild-type influenza infection.

Adverse Reactions/Side-effects (according to the package insert/patient information leaflet)

Very rare (may affect up to 1 in 1,000,000 people):
- severe allergic reaction: signs of a severe allergic reaction may include shortness of breath and swelling of the face or tongue.
- Guillain-Barré syndrome and exacerbation of symptoms of Leigh syndrome

Very common (may affect more than 1 in 10 people):
- runny or stuffy nose
- reduced appetite
- weakness
- headache

Common (may affect up to 1 in 10 people):
- fever
- muscle aches

Uncommon (may affect up to 1 in 100 people):
- rash
- nose bleed
- allergic reactions

Ingredients (according to the package insert/patient information leaflet)

Reassortant influenza virus* (live attenuated) of the following four strains**:
A/<Official strain> (H1N1)-like strain
(<actual strain>)107.0±0.5 FFU***

A/<Official strain> (H3N2)-like strain
(<actual strain>)107.0±0.5 FFU***

B/<Official strain> (Victoria lineage)-like strain
(<actual strain>)107.0±0.5 FFU***

B/<Official strain> (Yamagata lineage)-like strain
(<actual strain>)107.0±0.5 FFU***

per 0.2 ml dose

* propagated in fertilised hens' eggs from healthy chicken flocks.
** produced in VERO cells by reverse genetic technology. This product contains genetically

modified organisms (GMOs).
*** fluorescent focus units

The vaccine may contain residues of the following substances: egg proteins (e.g. ovalbumin) and gentamicin.

Sucrose
Dibasic potassium phosphate
Monobasic potassium phosphate
Gelatin (porcine, Type A)
Arginine hydrochloride
Monosodium glutamate monohydrate
Water for injections

References

1. Pediatr Infect Dis J. 2008 May;27(5):444-52
2. Pediatrics. 2005 Sep;116(3):e397-407
3. Pediatrics. 2002 Oct;110(4):662-72
4. Pedlatr Infect Dis J. 2004 Feb;23(2):138-44
5. Fluenz Tetra package insert
6. European Medicines Agency
7. National Vaccine Injury Compensation Program Statistics Report For January 2015

Gardasil

Manufacturer: Merck Sharp & Dohme Corp
Generic name: Human Papillomavirus Quadrivalent (Types 6, 11, 16, and 18) Vaccine, Recombinant

Gardasil Safety

With almost 30,000 adverse events reported to the US Vaccine Adverse Event Reporting System in only 9 years, HPV vaccines are the most controversial vaccine type of recent years. Safety concerns have led to the vaccine being withdrawn in Spain and Japan.
Merck says in its information that they conducted 7 clinical trials. In 5 out of 7, the placebo group received Amorphous Aluminum Hydroxyphosphate Sulfate (AAHS), the adjuvant used in Gardasil. One trial used a saline placebo and one was uncontrolled. In presenting the results, Merck compares adverse reaction from Gardasil to the placebo groups but does not always make clear whether that placebo group received saline solution or AAHS. Only for local "injection-site" reactions was this shown and Gardasil often had *many times* the adverse reactions than saline placebo – and so did AAHS. But for systemic adverse events, i.e. the important ones, they do not make clear whether they are comparing Gardasil to saline placebo or AAHS placebo.

In examining systemic *autoimmune* disorders, for example, the same percentage in both the vaccine and the placebo group had such adverse reaction but in this case we know that among the placebo recipients, only 4.5% received a saline placebo and the rest received Amorphous Aluminum Hydroxyphosphate Sulfate. The results are consequently highly misleading as they only show Gardasil being not much worse than its adjuvant alone. In addition, if the AAHS group had a higher incidence of a side-effect than the Gardasil group, then this side-effect was omitted from the data, which is indefensible.

Adverse events were recorded up to 14 days following injection of each dose. Merck says that "Of the entire study population (29,323 individuals), 0.04% of the reported serious systemic adverse reactions were judged to be vaccine related by the study investigator [i.e. themselves]."[1]

The vaccine was approved by the European Medicines Agency as "benefits outweigh the risks". [2] The NHS website concurs, saying "for most people the benefit of the vaccine far outweighs the risk", though it stops short of calling Gardasil safe. [3]

But in December 2014 a study found that Gardasil made it 5 times more likely to get Lupus, 4.6 times more likely to get gastroenteritis, 2.5 times more likely to get arthritis, 4 times more likely to get vasculitis, 1.8 times more likely to suffer Central Nervous System related problems and 8 times more likely to get alopecia as consequences of Serious Autoimmune Adverse Reactions, compared to controls.[4]

Gardasil Efficacy

According to the manufacturer's published data, almost everyone who receives a full course of Gardasil develops an immune response but they admit that they haven't established "duration of immunity". Their data shows the immunity wearing off within months, primarily in the age group targeted for vaccination. Antibody levels last well in the over 35s.

Merck also conducted several trials in which they tested whether Gardasil would prevent pre-cancerous lesions caused by high-risk HPV strains and they claim Gardasil is 100% effective in females aged 16-26 years who were not previously infected.[1] Efficacy was lower in other groups. They did not explain how this can be reconciled with the low duration of immunity.

This result sounds too good to be true but subsequent studies also found high efficacy using similar trial populations and similar outcome measures. A critique of the studies' design and data evaluation by different researchers can be found in the HPV chapter.

In order for Gardasil to be an effective cancer prevention, cervical cancer will have to turn out to be the only human cancer caused solely by a virus and Gardasil will have to prove long-term efficacy. But neither is the case so far.

Gardasil side-effects/adverse reactions (according to the package insert)

The most common side effects with GARDASIL are:
• pain, swelling, itching, bruising, and redness at the injection site
• headache
• fever
• nausea
• dizziness
• vomiting
• fainting

Other common side-effects are:
• Diarrhea
• Cough
• Toothache
• Upper respiratory tract infection
• Malaise
• Arthralgia
• Insomnia
• Nasal congestion

Gardasil contraindications (according to the package insert)

You should not get GARDASIL if you have, or have had:
• an allergic reaction after getting a dose of GARDASIL

- a severe allergic reaction to yeast, amorphous aluminum hydroxyphosphate sulfate, polysorbate 80

What should I tell my health care provider before getting GARDASIL?
Tell your health care provider if you:

- are pregnant or planning to get pregnant GARDASIL is not recommended for use in pregnant women
- have immune problems, like HIV infection, cancer, or you take medicines that affect your immune system
- have a fever over 100°F (37.8°C)
- had an allergic reaction to another dose of GARDASIL
- take any medicines, even those you can buy over the counter

Ingredients

- proteins of HPV Types 6, 11, 16, and 18
- amorphous aluminum hydroxyphosphate sulfate
- yeast protein
- sodium chloride
- L-histidine
- polysorbate 80
- sodium borate
- water for injection

References

1. Gardasil package insert/patient information leaflet
2. European Medicines Agency
3. NHS Website January2014
4. Clin Rheumatol. 2014 Dec 23.

Infanrix-IPV

Manufacturer: GlaxoSmithKline
Generic name: Diphtheria, tetanus, pertussis (acellular, component) and poliomyelitis (inactivated) vaccine (adsorbed)

Infanrix-IPV Safety

Safety assessment for Infanrix-IPV is based on studies done for its predecessor, Infanrix. The first was a small 335-infants study looking for pre-determined minor adverse events occurring within 3 days following vaccination. The study doesn't tell us much because a) it was too small and b) most parents aren't worried about short-term, minor side-effects. Two more studies in the US were of similar design and size but examined adverse reaction to Infanrix where this was used as a separate booster and not a primary course.[2]

Slightly more serious side-effects were looked for during the Italian efficacy trial, such as high fever, persistent crying of more than 3 hours and seizures. But no placebo was used. Instead, the effects were compared to that of another type of vaccine, namely a whole-cell DTP vaccine, which is notorious for its adverse reactions and which was replaced for this reason. Not surprisingly, Infanrix was much safer than this other vaccine.[2]

The only study which allowed for "unsolicited" adverse events, i.e. any side-effects and not just minor pre-selected ones, was the larger Germany study. [2] Unfortunately GlaxoSmithKline did not publish the full result in publicly available information and only gives some examples of minor events that happened within 7 days of any of the doses.

I have searched the US VAERS database (which is for adverse reactions that happened after a vaccines has been put into use) for the relevant vaccine types from this manufacturer (including the types for Infanrix and Infanrix-IPV). Serious events included convulsion, vomiting, hypotonia, cyanosis, diarrhoea and many others, including coma and death. The data doesn't necessarily mean that the vaccine was confirmed to be responsible, nor does it necessarily mean that these side-effects are very likely. But as only about 1-10% of vaccines adverse events are estimated to get reported as such, it is nevertheless important to mention these here. Of 12,000 total adverse events to date, over 2,000 have been classed as serious and 45 were classed as deaths. The total size of the database is around 200,000 events.[3]

Infanrix-IPV Efficacy

According to the manufacturer's information, trials involved around 1300 children and efficacy for each component of the vaccine (diphtheria, tetanus, whooping cough, polio) was established by measuring immunogenicity (antibody response). Pretty much anyone who received the vaccine had an antibody response considered adequate to provide protection. This was measured one month after injection/last dose. [1]

There is also reliance on studies which weren't for exactly this vaccine but for its predecessor, which is common practice. For the tetanus and diphtheria components, immunogenicity studies were again used. In all cases it was concluded that the vaccines is highly efficacious. [2] For the pertussis part, studies were carried out which actually looked at how many vaccine recipients got ill compared to non-vaccinated individuals (as opposed to only measuring immunogenicity). Only 285 individuals were part of the study and the results were markedly in favour of the vaccine being effective. [2] Had it been an independent study, this would be evidence in favour of Infanrix-IPV.

Adverse Reactions (according to the manufacturer)

Allergic reactions
If your child has an allergic reaction, see your doctor straight away. The signs may include:
- kin rashes that may be itchy or blistering
- swelling of the eyes and face
- difficulty in breathing or swallowing
- a sudden drop in blood pressure
- loss of consciousness

These signs usually start very soon after the injection has been given. Take your child to see a doctor straight away if they happen after leaving the clinic. Allergic reactions are very rare (less than 1 in 10,000 doses of the vaccine).

See your doctor straight away if your child has any of the following serious side effects:
- collapse
- loss of consciousness
- lack of awareness
- fits

See your doctor straight away if you notice any of the above. These side effects have happened with other vaccines against whooping cough. They usually occur within 2 to 3 days after vaccination.

Other side effects include:
Very common (these may occur with more than 1 in 10 doses of the vaccine):
- feeling sleepy
- headache
- loss of appetite
- high temperature of 38°C or higher
- pain, redness and swelling at the injection site
- unusual crying
- feeling irritable or restless

Common (these may occur with up to 1 in 10 doses of the vaccine):
- diarrhoea
- nausea
- vomiting (feeling or being sick)

- high temperature of 39.5°C or higher
- generally feeling unwell
- hard lump at the injection site
- feeling weak
- asthenia
- pruritis
- otitis media

Uncommon (these may occur with up to 1 in 100 doses of the vaccine):
- skin allergies or rash
- abdominal pain
- myalgia
- bronchitis

Rare (these may occur with up to 1 in 1,000 doses of the vaccine):
- swollen glands in the neck, armpit and groin (lymphadenopathy)
- coughing or chest infection (bronchitis)
- itching
- lumpy rash (hives).

Very rare (these may occur with up to 1 in 10,000 doses of the vaccine):
- bleeding or bruising more easily than normal (thrombocytopenia)
- temporarily stopping breathing (apnoea)
- swelling of the face, lips, mouth, tongue or throat which may cause difficulty in swallowing or breathing (angioneurotic oedema)
- blisters at the injection site

Contraindications (according to the manufacturer)

Infanrix-IPV should not be given if:
- your child is allergic (hypersensitive) to:
    - any of the ingredients in Infanrix-IPV
    - neomycin or polymyxin (types of antibiotics)
    - formaldehyde.
    Signs of an allergic reaction may include itchy skin rash, shortness of breath and swelling of the face or tongue.

- your child has had an allergic reaction to any vaccine against diphtheria, tetanus, whooping cough or polio
- your child experienced problems of the nervous system (encephalopathy) within 7 days after previous vaccination with a vaccine against whooping cough
- your child has a severe infection with a high temperature (over 38°C). A minor infection such as a cold should not be a problem, but talk to your doctor first.

Infanrix-IPV should not be given if any of the above apply to your child. If you are not sure, talk to your doctor or pharmacist before your child is given Infanrix-IPV.

Take special care with Infanrix-IPV:
Check with your doctor or pharmacist before your child is given this vaccine if:

- after previously having Infanrix-IPV or another vaccine against whooping cough, your child had any problems, especially:
    - ~ a high temperature (over 40°C) within 48 hours of vaccination
    - ~ a collapse or "shock-like" state within 48 hours of vaccination
    - ~ persistent crying lasting 3 hours or more within 48 hours of vaccination
    - ~ fits with or without a high temperature within 3 days of vaccination

- your child is suffering from an undiagnosed or progressive disease of the brain or uncontrolled epilepsy. After control of the disease the vaccine should be administered.
- your child has a bleeding problem or bruises easily
- your child has a tendency to fits due to a fever or if there is a history in the family of this
- your child has problems with their immune system (including HIV infection). Your child may still be given Infanrix-IPV. However, the protection against the infections may not be as high.

Ingredients

The active substances are:
- Diphtheria toxoid(1)
- Tetanus toxoid(1)
- Bordetella pertussis antigens
- Pertussis toxoid(1)
- Filamentous Haemagglutinin(1)
- Pertactin(1)
- Poliovirus (inactivated)(2) type 1 (Mahoney strain) type 2 (MEF-1 strain) type 3 (Saukett strain)

(1) adsorbed on aluminium hydroxide, hydrated
(2) propagated in VERO cells

The other ingredients are:
- sodium chloride
- Medium 199 (containing principally amino acids, mineral salts, vitamins)
- water for injections.

References

1. Infanrix-IPV patient information leaflet/package insert
2. Infanrix package insert
3. http://wonder.cdc.gov/vaers.html

Meningitec

Manufacturer: Wyeth Pharmaceuticals
Generic name: Meningococcal Group C Conjugate Vaccine

Meningitec Safety

All safety studies were small and short term. Adverse effects were only counted as vaccine-related if they happened 2 – 3 days following injection and only minor, local side-effects were looked for. About the worst side-effects that were looked for were vomiting (up to 12% of infants) and fever above 38ºC (up to 9% of infants). Where serious side-effects were mentioned, these were 3 cases out of a group of 124 in one trial (bowel obstruction, bronchitis/pneumonia and fever of 40ºC) and 5 out of 106 in another trial (but including some which happened up to a month after the injection and could be unrelated, including high fevers, seizures and pneumonia). The only larger safety study (of 2877 infants) recorded 5 sudden infant deaths in the meningitec group and 4 in that of another vaccine. [1] There is no evidence that the vaccines caused these, although if the UK average was used, we would only expect to see around 0.17 – 0.3 sudden infant deaths for this size of group. [2,3] In other words the risk of sudden infant death would be 30-times higher after receiving the vaccine. Whether this is a fair comparison or not is of course uncertain. The trial participants may, by chance, have had a higher proportion of other risk factors.

The UK regulator's "yellow card" scheme collected 14,000 reports relating to this type of vaccine over the last 15 years, including 37 deaths, but these cases are not confirmed to have been caused by the vaccine. A report can be submitted by anyone who thinks that a drug caused a side-effect.

Meningitec Efficacy

The UK medicines regulator, the MHRA, states in its public assessment report for Meningitec: "The clinical efficacy section of this application is based on demonstration of adequate immunogenicity. Efficacy studies have not been performed". They say this is justified based on already licensed vaccines being similar. They also say that it would be impractical to do a proper trial, as it would have to involve the entire UK child population. They do not say why this should be so, but a possible explanation is that the benefits of vaccinating against meningococcal infections are so minor, that it would take that many trial subjects in order to see any positive results. Lastly they claim that there was an established link between immunogenicity (antibody response from the vaccine) and protection against disease, based on the Hib vaccine.[1]

The UK medicines regulator MHRA states "This was the first application for a conjugate meningococcal serogroup C vaccine in any country (EU and non-EU)", which appears to invalidated the above justifications for not needing efficacy trials at least to some extend.

The entire approval process is, as always, based on data supplied by the manufacturer. In trying to prove that the vaccine causes an adequate antibody response in patients, they supplied data from various "immunogenicity trials", 7 of which related to infants. These were small studies, usually involving fewer than 100 patients. Immunogenicity does not really equate to protection but the trials studied nothing else. They compared the antibody response of Meningitec to other vaccines in order to establish that the results are at least as good. Although they found the levels of immunogenicity they were looking for, the effect wore off in less than a year. A booster using a different type of vaccine was used to fix this problem but instead of presenting the whole data, the source document only picked 40 subjects, presumably those whose results were favourable, and presented only that data, and only with a follow-up time of 4 weeks. Among the 40 infants whose data was presented, everyone had the looked-for antibody levels 4 weeks after the booster.[1]

Overall there appears to be no evidence that vaccinated children are protected against meningococcal infections, let alone that the vaccine reduces incidents of meningitis.

Meningitec side-effects/adverse reactions (according to the package insert)

The following are taken from the manufacturers patient information leaflet. They will not include all side-effects and may not include the most serious ones.

Mild Effects
- local reaction around the injection site such as redness, itchiness, tenderness, pain or discomfort, warmth, burning or stinging, swelling or the formation of hard lumps or scars
- headache
- aching muscles
- dizziness and light-headedness
- sleepiness or unsettled sleep
- generally feeling unwell or irritability
- unusual high-pitched crying
- eating and drinking less than usual, loss of appetite
- diarrhoea or vomiting
- stomach cramps or pain
- heartburn
- fever

Other very rare side effects include:
- swollen glands in the neck, armpits or groin
- pins and needles
- loss of muscle tone
- decreased sensitivity to touch

Serious Effects
If any of the following happen, tell your doctor or pharmacist immediately or go to Accident and Emergency at your nearest hospital:
- sudden signs of allergy such as rash, itching or hives on the skin, swelling of the face, lips, tongue or other parts of the body
- red or purple flat pinhead spots or bruising appear under the skin

- shortness of breath, wheezing or trouble breathing, chest pain
- temporarily stopping breathing
- a seizure (fit) or convulsion, which may be accompanied by a very high temperature
- feeling weak or paralysed, or generally feeling sore or tender
- dark coloured urine or pale stools
- relapse of a kidney condition called nephrotic syndrome.

Meningitec contraindications (according to the package insert)

- allergic reactions to the vaccine or any ingredients
- blood/bleeding disorders
- conditions that lower immunity
- infections or high fever

Ingredients

Active ingredients:
Each vial contains 10 micrograms meningococcal Group C oligosaccharide conjugated to 15 micrograms of diphtheria CRM197 protein.
Other ingredients:
- Aluminium phosphate
- Sodium chloride
- Water for injections

References

1. MHRA Public Assessment Report, Meningitec Meningococcal serogroup C oligosaccharide conjugate vaccine (adsorbed), UK/H/0356/02/DC UK licence no: PL 00011/0496, John Wyeth & Brother Limited
2. UNICEF website accessed May 2014
3. Office of National Statistics website access January 2014

Menitorix

Manufacturer: GlaxoSmithKline
Generic Name: Haemophilus influenzae type b and Meningococcal group C conjugate vaccine

Menitorix Safety

Menitorix was co-administered in various trials with other vaccines. The manufacturer says "There was no evidence that the reactions other than injection site reactions were related to Menitorix rather than the concomitant vaccine." [1] I find this rather unhelpful. A proper placebo group did not exist and it appears that there is also no evidence that the side-effects were *not* caused by Menitorix. They simply don't know, which is not surprising, if one co-administers other vaccines at the same time.

The UK reporting system for adverse reactions recorded 244 reports for this type of vaccine over the last 8 years, with 4 deaths, including some from the diseases which the vaccine is meant to protect from. These numbers are very low and they do not prove that the vaccine was to blame for all or even any of the reported reactions. However, considering that vaccine adverse reactions are thought to be widely under-reported, it seems fair at least to mention those that did get reported.

Certainly the now common practice of injecting different vaccines at the same time and then saying "there was no evidence it was *our* vaccine that cause the side-effects" points to a very worrying disregard for safety among vaccine manufacturers.

Menitorix Efficacy

Menitorix is a combined Men C and Hib vaccine and was tested for efficacy using immunogenicity trials. They compared antibody response in subjects receiving Menitorix with those from comparable vaccines to establish that Menitorix is non-inferior, i.e. at least as good as existing vaccines. They found that almost everyone had the looked-for antibody density but also, as with many vaccines, that this wore off quickly. After one year, there was "clear evidence of waning protection." A booster given one year after the "primary course" is supposed to fix this problem and according to the manufacturer, everyone who received this booster had good antibody density 18 months after injection. [1] This appears to be the longest follow-up period considered, which the manufacturer presented as "long-term persistence" data.

Immunogenicity (antibody response) is a poor substitute for proper efficacy trials and does not tell us if the child in question will get ill or not. Infectious disease have very often been found to break out in populations with high vaccination coverage and where individuals had "protective" antibody counts.

Contraindications (according to the package insert)

Menitorix should not be given:

- if your child previously had any allergic reaction to Menitorix, to any Hib or MenC vaccine, to tetanus toxoid or to any other ingredients of this medicine (listed in section 6). Signs of an allergic reaction may include itchy skin rash, shortness of breath and swelling of the face or tongue.
- if your child has a high temperature (38oC or above) or a severe infection. It is usual to wait until the child is better before giving the vaccine. A minor infection such as a cold should not be a problem but talk to your doctor or nurse first.

Remember that the first dose of Menitorix should not be given before your child is 2 months of age.

Warnings and precautions
Talk to your doctor or nurse before your child receives Menitorix
- if your child has a bleeding problem or bruises easily.
- if your child takes medicines or has any treatment which may affect the immune system. Also, if your child has HIV infection or any other illness that can reduce his or her immunity to infections. Your child can still be given Menitorix if your doctor or nurse advises it but your child may not develop as good protection against Hib and MenC infections as other children.
- if your child was born prematurely (before 37 weeks). Menitorix can be given from the age of 2 months after birth onwards but it is not known if protection against Hib and MenC will be as good as in children born at term.

Side-effects/adverse reactions (according to the package insert)

The following are taken from the manufacturers patient information leaflet. They will not necessarily include all side-effects and may not include the most serious ones.

Very common (these may occur with more than 1 in 10 doses of the vaccine):
- Pain, redness or swelling at the site of the injection
- Fever (temperature of 38C or above)
- Irritability
- Loss of appetite
- Sleepiness

Common (these may occur with up to 1 in 10 doses of the vaccine):
- Injection site reaction, such as hard lump

Uncommon (these may occur with up to 1 in 100 doses of the vaccine):
- Crying
- Diarrhoea
- Being sick
- Skin allergies
- Fever more than 39.5°C
- Rash

Rare (these may occur with up to 1 in 1,000 doses of the vaccine):
• Abdominal pain
• Sleeplessness
• Generally feeling unwell

Unknown frequency
• Lymphadenopathy
• Febrile seizures
• Hypotonia
• Headache
• Dizziness
• Allergic reactions (including urticaria and anaphylactoid reactions)

References
1. Menitorix product information

Menjugate

Manufacturer: Novartis
Generic Name: Neisseria Meningitidis Group C Capsular Polysaccharide Protein Conjugate

Menjugate Safety

In order to assess the safety profile of the vaccine, the manufacturer divided trial participants into age groups and administered Menjugate together with other vaccines. Solicited (meaning pre-determined) adverse events were then recorded up to 7 days following vaccination. Of course, with this trial design, it is later impossible to know which vaccine caused a certain adverse reaction and that is intentional. It allows the manufacturer to say that there is no evidence that it was their vaccine which was responsible and that it could have been the other vaccine.
That is exactly what happened here. A proper placebo control group would be a very easy way of finding out the truth, which is why placebo groups are rarely used. The adverse events that are presented in the product information were numerous and the risk varied from study to study. As an example, diarrhoea occurred in up to 43% of babies, vomiting in up to 34%, high fever in up to 9% and irritability in up to 81%. But exactly which vaccine caused these remains unknown.[1]

Novartis were honest enough to publish serious adverse reactions which had been reported once the vaccine was in wider use and they classified most of them as "very rare" (e.g. lymphadenopathy, anaphylaxis, seizures, photophobia, myalgia). They say they divided the number of reports by the number of doses distributed, to arrive at how frequently these reactions occurred. [1] This does not take into account the problem of under-reporting and although it could be argued that under-reporting is not the manufacturer's problem when presenting data, it is nevertheless very real and contorts the data. Many more serious adverse events could be added. The MHRA, the UK's regulator, recorded over 14,000 adverse events and 37 deaths since 1999 from vaccines of this kind. The MHRA data only shows that someone believed the vaccine to be responsible for a certain side-effect. It doesn't prove that the vaccine was responsible, nor does it help evaluate the likelihood. But as most vaccine-related adverse reactions are never reported in the first place, it is nevertheless fair to report those cases that have.

Menjugate Efficacy

The manufacturer's own information [1] states:
"As shown in clinical trials, Menjugate is highly immunogenic [4,5] and induces protective levels of bactericidal antibodies [6-8] in a significant number of subjects after vaccination. [9,11,13]"

I researched the referenced material. [4] relates to a publication which discusses a new technique of measuring antibodies and [5] discusses the problem of different measuring techniques being used in different laboratories. Neither was intended to prove if Menjugate works. [5] does refer to other studies which are supposed to have shown increased antibody counts following vaccination, but the authors are in fact cautious about the meaning of this and point out that no efficacy trials have been done to show that there is a protective effect from it.

[6] is entirely unrelated. [7] is a 1969 paper examining the link between antibodies and "susceptibility". It doesn't relate to the vaccine at all, which it precedes by decades, and in fact points out that antibodies can't be the only factor in protecting a person. "Indeed, there is no evidence that humoral antibodies are the sole, or even the major host defense mechanism." I could not find [8].

[9,11] are studies comparing immunogenicity of different types of vaccine and [13] is the same as [11]. These studies do suggest that the conjugate type vaccines, of which Menjugate is one, have an immunogenic effect.
The manufacturer refers to another study in particular relating to infants [2]. This study also measured immunogenicity (in fairly small groups), comparing different vaccines, and favouring the conjugate type vaccine.

In summary, I'm not aware of Novartis having offered any evidence that Menjugate works. Some of the studies referenced show that similar vaccines cause an antibody response but not whether recipients of the vaccine are less likely to get ill. The remaining studies are either unrelated or do not support the claims made by Novartis. One even contradicts them. It can only be assumed that they hoped no one would read the referenced material.

Menjugate Contraindications (according to the package insert)

• allergy to the active substance or any of the other ingredients of Menjugate Kit
• allergy to diphtheria toxoid
• allergy following vaccination with Menjugate Kit in the past
• very high fever

The manufacturer has also stated the following:

"Although symptoms of meningism such as neck pain/stiffness or photophobia have been reported, there is no evidence that the vaccine causes meningococcal C meningitis."

"Any acute infection or febrile illness is reason for delaying the use of Menjugate except when, in the opinion of the physician, withholding the vaccine entails a greater risk. A minor afebrile illness, such as a mild upper respiratory infection, is not usually reason to defer immunization."

"The tip cap of the diluent syringe contains 10% Dry Natural Rubber. Although the risk for developing allergic latex reactions is very small, healthcare professionals are encouraged to consider the benefit risk prior to administering this vaccine to patients with known history of hypersensitivity to latex."

"The vaccine should not be used during pregnancy unless there is defined risk of meningococcal C disease, in which case the risk-benefit ratio should be evaluated."
"The effect on breast-fed infants of the administration of Menjugate to their mothers has not been studied."

"There are no data in adults aged 65 years and older."

Side-effects/adverse reactions (according to the package insert)

The following are taken from the manufacturers patient information leaflet. They will not necessarily include all side-effects and may not include the most serious ones.

The most common side effects reported during clinical trials usually lasted only one to two days and were not usually severe. The side effects were:

Very common (in more than 1 in 10 people):
• Redness, swelling and tenderness/pain at the injection site
• Vomiting
• Irritability
• Drowsiness
• Difficulty sleeping
• Loss of appetite and diarrhea

Common (less than 1 in 10 people):
• Fever
• Crying

Very rare (less than 1 in 10,000 people):
• Enlarged lymph glands
• Dizziness
• Faints
• Numbness
• Tingling sensation or pins and needles
• Temporarily reduced muscle tone
• Visual disturbances and sensitivity to light

Ingredients (per dose)

• 10 micrograms of Neisseria meningitidis group C (strain C11) oligosaccharide chemically joined to 12.5 to 25.0 micrograms of Corynebacterium diphtheriae CRM197 protein
• aluminium hydroxide (0.3 to 0.4 mg Al3+)
• mannitol
• sodium dihydrogen phosphate monohydrate
• disodium phosphate heptahydrate
• sodium chloride
• water

References

1 Menjugate Product Monograph
2 JAMA. 2000 Jun 7;283(21):2795-801
4 Clin Diagn Lab Immunol. Jul 1998; 5(4): 479–485
5 Clin Diagn Lab Immunol. Mar 1997; 4(2): 156–167
6 J Infect Dis. 1995 Nov;172(5):1279-89
7 J Exp Med. 1969 Jun 1;129(6):1307-26
9 Vaccine. 2000 Jun 1;18(24):2686-92
11 JAMA. 1998 Nov 18;280(19):1685-9

MMRVaxPro

Manufacturer: Sanofi Pasteur MSD
Generic name: Measles, mumps and rubella vaccine (live)

MMRVaxPro Safety

Sanofi Pasteur says that MMRVaxPro has a similar safety profile to a predecessor vaccine, implying that this means it must be safe. They also recorded adverse reactions to MMRVaxPro in 1,940 children (they omitted any that happened to fewer than 4 children, which they call "isolated reports" (I would comment that 4 children out of 1,940 still matter) and found mainly minor side-effects. Among the more serious ones were aseptic meningitis, encephalitis and encephalopathy, subacute sclerosing panencephalitis, arthralgia and arthritis. However, they stress that either the vaccine wasn't proven to be the cause or else that they were very rare events.[1]

The UK Yellow Card scheme has recorded over 8,000 reports and 28 deaths relating to MMR vaccines but this data covers a 27 year period and there is no certainty that the vaccines really caused these fatalities. Yet conversely, under-reporting means that the true incidence rate could be one hundred times higher. 9 out of the 38 fatalities were recorded simply as death, sudden death or sudden infant death. It is not unreasonable to suggest that the vast majority of SIDs will never be reported as vaccine related, even if they happened soon after vaccination.

On the US VAERS database, MMR vaccines make up 15% of the entire database of adverse reactions. Most of them were classed as "not serious". 324 were for deaths and over 1000 each for "life threatening" or "permanent disability". Once again this data does not prove that vaccines were responsible in all cases but neither does it reflect the true number of cases due to under-reporting. It only tells us that MMR vaccines are one of the most reported vaccine types on the database.

MMRVaxPro Efficacy

According to the manufacturer, MMRVaxPro was compared in a study to another MMR vaccine and found to be similar in immunogenicity. In other words, both vaccines produced an antibody response. They also present data for the other MMR vaccine, proving its immunogenicity. So far I have no reason to doubt any of this Most vaccines manage to elicit an immune response in form of antibodies (immunogenicity) and there is no reason to doubt that these vaccines did the same. However, they also refer to field trials which they say showed that the immunogenicity "paralleled protection from these diseases".

This is the really interesting bit, namely whether the recipients of the vaccine were less likely to get ill. Immunogenicity alone does not automatically prove this.
I could not identify the trial referred to from the information provided but there is ample data available that shows MMR recipients are much less likely to get measles (see for example [?]). At the same time there is also amply evidence for the opposite, namely outbreaks where most

children who got ill were in fact fully vaccinated (see chapters on Measles, Mumps and Rubella). One possible explanation is waning immunity. If the vaccines protect children for a short while, then this would produce good results in studies looking at young children who got vaccinated fairly recently, while older children would still get ill.

MMRVaxPro Contraindications (according to the package insert)

Do not use M-M-RVAXPRO:
- If you or your child are allergic to any of the components of this vaccine (including neomycin or any of the other ingredients
- If you or your child are pregnant (in addition, pregnancy should be avoided for 1 month after vaccination)
- If you or your child have any illness with fever higher than 38.5°C; however, low-grade fever itself is not a reason to delay vaccination
- If you or your child have active untreated tuberculosis
- If you or your child have a blood disorder or any type of cancer that affects the immune system
- If you or your child are receiving treatment or taking medicines that may weaken the immune system (except low-dose corticosteroid therapy for asthma or replacement therapy)
- If you or your child have a weakened immune system because of a disease (including AIDS)
- If you or your child have a family history of congenital or hereditary immunodeficiency, unless the immune competence of your or your child is demonstrated.

Warnings and precaution
Talk to the doctor or pharmacist before you or your child receive M-M-RVAXPRO if you have experienced any of the following:
- If you or your child have an allergic reaction to eggs or anything that contained egg
- If you or your child have a history or family history of allergies or of convulsions (fits)
- If you or your child have a side effect after vaccination with measles, mumps, or rubella vaccine (in a single component vaccine or a combined vaccine, such as the measles, mumps, and rubella vaccine manufactured by Merck & Co., Inc., or M-M-RVAXPRO) that involved easy bruising or bleeding for longer than usual
- If you or your child have infection with Human Immunodeficiency Virus (HIV) but do not show symptoms of HIV disease. You or your child should be monitored closely for measles, mumps, and rubella because vaccination may be less effective than for uninfected persons.

MMRVaxPro side-effects/adverse reactions (according to the package insert)

The following are taken from the manufacturers patient information leaflet. They will not necessarily include all side-effects and may not include the most serious ones.
Very common (may affect more than 1 in 10):
- Fever (38.5°C or higher)
- Injection-site redness; injection-site pain; injection-site swelling

Common (may affect 1 to 10 in 100):
- Rash (including measles-like rash)

- Injection-site bruising

Uncommon (may affect 1 to 10 in 1000):
- Nasal congestion and sore throat; upper respiratory tract infection or viral infection; runny nose
- Diarrhoea, vomiting
- Hives
- Injection-site rash

Not known (Frequency cannot be estimated from the available data):
- Aseptic meningitis (fever, feeling sick, vomiting, headache, stiff neck, and sensitivity to light); swollen testicles; infection of the middle ear; inflamed salivary glands; atypical measles (described in patients who received a killed measles virus vaccine, usually given before 1975)
- Swollen lymph nodes
- Bruising or bleeding more easily than normal
- Severe allergic reaction that may include difficulty in breathing, facial swelling, localised swelling, and swelling of the limbs
- Irritability
- Seizures (fits) without fever; seizures (fits) with fever in children; walking unsteadily; dizziness; illnesses involving inflammation of the nervous system (brain and/or spinal cord)
- An illness consisting of muscle weakness, abnormal sensations, tingling in the arms, legs, and upper body (Guillain-Barré syndrome)
- Headache; fainting; nerve disorders which can cause weakness, tingling, or numbness; eye nerve disturbances
- Discharge and itching of the eyes with crusting of eyelids (conjunctivitis)
- Inflammation of the retina (in the eye) with changes in sight
- Deafness
- Cough; lung infection with or without fever
- Feeling sick (nausea)
- Itching; inflammation of the fatty tissue under the skin; red or purple, flat, pinhead spots under the skin; hardened, raised area of the skin; serious illness with ulcers or blistering of the skin, mouth, eyes, and/or genitals (Stevens-Johnson syndrome)
- Joint pain and/or swelling (usually transient and rarely chronic); muscle pain
- Burning and/or stinging of short duration at the injection site; blisters and/or hives at the injection site
- Generally feeling unwell (malaise); swelling; soreness
- Inflammation of blood vessels

Ingredients

The active substances are:
- Measles virus(1) Enders' Edmonston strain (live, attenuated)
- Mumps virus(1) Jeryl Lynn™ [Level B] strain (live, attenuated)
- Rubella virus(2) Wistar RA 27/3 strain (live, attenuated)

(1) produced in chick embryo cells.
(2) produced in WI-38 human diploid lung fibroblasts.

The other ingredients are:
- sorbitol
- sodium phosphate
- potassium phosphate
- sucrose
- hydrolysed gelatin
- medium 199 with Hanks' salts
- MEM
- monosodium L-glutamate
- neomycin
- phenol red
- sodium bicarbonate
- hydrochloric acid (to adjust pH)
- sodium hydroxide (to adjust pH)
- water for injections

References

1. MMRVaxPro Summery of Product Characteristics
2. Pediatr Infect Dis J. 1999 Jul;18(7):620-3

NeisVac-C

Manufacturer: Baxter
Generic name: Meningococcal Group C Polysaccharide Conjugate Vaccine Adsorbed

NeisVac-C Safety

The vaccine was tested, as has become common practice, in trials that administered other vaccines at the same time. Mostly they studied how likely "solicited" events were to occur, which means that it was decided beforehand, which minor side-effects to look out for and record. [1] As a consequence, other side-effects can go unreported. In addition, the manufacturer of the trial vaccine will be able to say that there was no evidence that their vaccine was to blame for any of the side-effects, rather than one of the other vaccines administered at the same time. It was already unsatisfactory when vaccine safety trials were done without a real placebo group, where the control group was another vaccine. Now the trials have become even more meaningless. The list further below contains the adverse reactions which were found and published.

Like many vaccines, NeisVac-C contains aluminium hydroxide, a widely-used adjuvant in vaccines. Previous mercury-containing adjuvants are now less common and it is hoped that those based on aluminium are safer. But due to the lack of long-term studies, we have to rely on passive reporting of vaccine adverse reactions, which usually tell us very little about the real risk. Whether or not the new adjuvants are safe is questionable. They are both strongly attacked and strongly defended. Safety levels are arbitrary and the effect on infants and their developing bodies (especially neurologically) is unknown.

The MHRA, the UK's regulator, recorded over 14,000 adverse events and 37 deaths since 1999 from vaccines of this kind. The MHRA data only shows that someone believed the vaccine to be responsible for a certain side-effect. It doesn't prove that the vaccine was responsible, nor does it help evaluate the likelihood. It is offered here nevertheless for reference.

NeisVac-C Efficacy

Baxter presented data showing that NeisVac-C is highly immunogenic, meaning that in almost everyone it causes an antibody response that is thought to be protective. They admitted that the effect lasts less than one year. Antibody titers went up again following a booster dose, but there was no further follow-up longer than about one month after the booster.

Baxter were honest enough to also admit that experience from the UK vaccination programme showed "there was clear evidence of waning protection" after one year. However they also say that NeisVac-C was exclusively used for meningococcal vaccinations in the Netherlands and that a sharp decrease had been recorded in meningococcal C diseases since.

They conclude: "Formal protective efficacy studies have not been performed." [1]

NeisVac-C Contraindications (according to the package insert)

Do not use NeisVac-C
- if you have ever had an allergic reaction to a previous dose of this vaccine or to any ingredient of the vaccine including tetanus toxoid. The symptoms of an allergic reaction include skin rash, swelling of the face and throat, difficulty in breathing, blue discolouration of the tongue or lips, low blood pressure, and collapse.
- if you have ever had an allergic reaction to any other vaccine intended to protect against meningococcal group C infections.

Vaccination with NeisVac-C may have to be delayed if you have an infectious illness (for example, high temperature, sore throat, cough, cold or flu). In this case, your doctor may advise you to postpone your vaccination until you are better.

Take special care with NeisVac-C
- if you have haemophilia or any other problem that may stop your blood from clotting properly
- if you have been told that you have an autoimmune disease or that you have a weak immune system for any reason. For example: Have you been told that you do not produce antibodies very efficiently? Are you taking medicines that reduce your immunity to infections (such as anti-cancer drugs or high doses of corticosteroids)?
- if you have had your spleen removed or have been told that your spleen does not work as it should
- if you suffer from a kidney disease in which large amounts of protein appear in the urine (called nephrotic syndrome) There have been reports that this condition may reappear after vaccination. Your doctor will advise you if you can still have NeisVac-C. What he says will depend on the exact type of kidney problem you have.
- if you are over 65 years old.

In these cases, talk to your doctor before receiving this vaccine, as it may not be suitable for you. You may still be given the vaccine but it may not provide very high protection against infections caused by the group C bacteria.
This medicinal product contains less than 1 mmol sodium (23 milligrams) per dose, i.e. essentially "sodium-free".

NeisVac-C Adverse reactions (according to the package insert)

The following are taken from the manufacturers patient information leaflet. They will not necessarily include all side-effects and may not include the most serious ones.

The following side effects have been reported:
Very common side effects (affect more than 1 in 10 people)
In all age groups:
- Redness, swelling, tenderness, and pain at the site of injection
- Headache

In infants and / or toddlers:
- Loss of appetite
- Feeling or being sick
- Diarrhoea
- Crying
- Irritability
- Drowsiness
- Sleepiness
- Poor sleep

In older children:
- Pains in the arms or legs

Common side effects (affect less than 1 in 10 people)
In all age groups:
- Fever

In children:
- Loss of appetite
- Feeling or being sick
- Diarrhoea
- Pains in the arms or legs

In adults and older children:
Muscle pain

The following side effects have also been reported:

- Skin rashes that can cover much of the body and lead to blistering and peeling. The inside of the mouth and the eyes can also be affected.
- Itching
- Hives
- Other rashes
- Swollen lymph glands
- Dizziness
- Fainting
- Abnormal or reduced sensation
- Loss of muscle tone or floppiness in infants
- Purple spots or blotches under the skin, which may be caused by a drop in special blood cells responsible for clotting. This may look like bruising.
- Fits (seizures) – These include reports of some fits in people who already suffered occasional fits. In teenagers and adults, some of the reports of fits may actually have been fainting attacks. In infants and young children, fits were usually associated with fever and were likely to be febrile convulsions. Most people recovered rapidly after the fit.

Ingredients

One dose (0.5 millilitres) of the vaccine consists of

- 10 micrograms of Neisseria meningitidis group C (strain 11) polysaccharide (de-O-acetylated)
- Tetanus toxoid
- Hydrated aluminium hydroxide (0.5 milligrams Al3+).
- Sodium chloride (cooking salt)
- Water

References

1. NeisVac-C product monograph

Pediacel

Manufacturer: Sanofi Pasteur MSD Limited
Generic name: Diphtheria, tetanus, pertussis (acellular, component), poliomyelitis (inactivated) and Haemophilus type b conjugate vaccine (adsorbed)

Pediacel Safety

Pediacel safety trials were small-scale and short-term and only compared adverse reaction to other vaccines. All trials were conducted by the manufacturer, who was in full control of which data to include in the study or present to the regulators.

Side-effects recorded since the vaccine was approved can be very serious. They include meningitis, convulsion, encephalopathy, SIDS and sudden death. The number of such adverse reactions reported are very low. For example the FDA, in a 2008 review, mentioned 14 deaths over a period of 9 years. However, vaccine side-effects are widely under-reported and only data forwarded by the manufacturer was analysed in this FDA review.

The vaccine contains a number of toxic ingredients, including Aluminim phospate, a neurotoxin, Phenoxyethanol, a reproductive toxin and Polysorbate 80, which can cause severe non-immunologic anaphylactoid reactions.

During the time of the previous DPT vaccine there was widespread concern over the amount of patients suffering serious side-effects [3,5], incl. neurological damage, following vaccination. Several studies found a link [12,13], while others found no link [7] or were inconclusive [6,9]. The vaccine was also suspected of increasing the likelihood of asthma later on in childhood. [10] One study found those links too but then adjusted the data [11] after which there was no link. Both sides of the argument accused each other of using data selectively and studies can be found "proving" either side of the argument. In most cases, only those children who showed symptoms within 7 days of vaccination were included in studies.
The problem was the pertussis part of the vaccine, which one can obviously not avoid in a combined vaccine.

Pediacel is a different type of vaccine and uses an acellular instead of a whole cell pertussis component. The hope is that the side effects will be less severe and less common and the data supports this so far [1,2,4,8]. But considering its scandal hit predecessor, extensive safety studies should have been conducted before licensing the vaccine.

Pediacel Efficacy

Clinical trials conducted by the manufacturer measured immunogenicity of Pediacel compared to other vaccines. They used 3 doses, each one month apart, and another dose about a year later. Immunogenicity was measured one month after dose 3 and 4, which means they tested for the presence of antibodies in the blood of the trial subjects. These results were positive and showed the hoped for density of antibodies per ml of blood.

It is often assumed that a certain amount of antibodies means the vaccines is effective and has given the patient immunity. This assumption has however long been disproved. In addition, measuring for antibodies only one month after the last dose is a very short time and does not help understand long-term efficacy. While the trials may prove an immune response to the vaccine itself, they do not prove anything about whether vaccinated people will be less likely to get ill.

In terms of measuring the vaccines ability to actually protect against contracting any of the 5 diseases it is meant to protect from, meaning a trial that actually looks at how many people get ill, only evidence on pertussis (whooping cough) was presented. The relevant trials are referred to as the Swedish efficacy trials and tested the efficacy of different pertussis vaccines compared to each other. [14] Pediacel was not tested as such but one vaccine was similar to Pediacel. The results are presented as positive but there was no real placebo group. Unless we compare the rate to an unvaccinated population, we simply cannot know if the vaccine prevented illness.

It may sound reasonable that a 5 in 1 vaccine should not have to "reinvent the wheel" by proving itself again for all the individual components, which have been tested in the past. But with almost all vaccine efficacy trials being based on immunogenicity only or else on comparison with other vaccines, there is no basis on which to base a claim of efficacy.

Pediacel side-effects/adverse reactions (according to the package insert)

The following are taken from the manufacturers patient information leaflet. They will not include all side-effects and may not include the most serious ones.

Reported side-effects (adverse reactions):

Very common (≥1/10):
- Appetite loss
- Irritability, Abnormal crying
- Vomiting
- Decreased activity, injection site tenderness, injection site erythema, pyrexia (≥38°C), injection site swelling

Common (≥1/100 to <1/10):
- Diarrhoea
- Injection site bleeding, injection site bruising

Uncommon (≥1/1,000 to <1/100):
- Extensive limb swelling (from the injection site beyond one or both
- joints)
- Convulsion (with or without fever)

Rare: None

Very Rare: None

Unknown frequency:
- Hypersensitivity, anaphylactic reaction (such as urticaria, angioedema)
- High-pitched crying, hypotonic hyporesponsive episode (infant appears pale, hypotonic (limp) and unresponsive)
- Pallor
- Rash
- Pain in vaccinated limb
- Pyrexia (>40.5°C), injection site mass, asthenia, and listlessness.

Pediacel contraindications (according to the package insert)

PEDIACEL should not be administered to children with known hypersensitivity
- to diphtheria, tetanus, pertussis, polio or Hib vaccines
- to any other component of the vaccine
- to any residual substances carried over from manufacture (neomycin, streptomycin, polymyxin B, glutaraldehyde, formaldehyde and bovine serum albumin), which may be present in undetectable trace amounts.

PEDIACEL is contraindicated if the infant has experienced an encephalopathy of unknown aetiology, occurring within 7 days following previous vaccination with pertussis containing vaccine. In these circumstances pertussis vaccination should be discontinued and the vaccination course should be continued with diphtheria, tetanus, polio and Hib vaccines.

Progressive neurologic disorder, including infantile spasms, uncontrolled epilepsy, progressive encephalopathy. Pertussis vaccine should not be administered to children with such conditions until a treatment regimen has been established and the condition has stabilized.

As with other vaccines, administration of PEDIACEL should be postponed in children suffering from acute severe febrile illness. The presence of a minor infection (e.g., mild upper respiratory infection) is not a contraindication.

Ingredients

Active Ingredients:
- Diphtheria Toxoid
- Tetanus Toxoid
- Acellular Pertussis Antigens
- Filamentous Haemagglutinin (FHA)
- Pertactin (PRN)
- Fimbriae Types 2 and 3 (FIM)
- Poliovirus (Inactivated)
    - ~ Type 1 (Mahoney)

~ Type 2 (MEF-1)

~ Type 3 (Saukett)

• Haemophilus influenzae Type b Polysaccharide (Polyribosylribitol Phosphate) Conjugated to Tetanus Toxoid (PRP-T)

Other Ingredients:

• Aluminim phospate (1.5 mg / 0.33mg aluminium)

• Phenoxyethanol

• Polysorbate 80

References

1. Dev Biol Stand. 1997;89:83-9
2. Cochrane Database Syst Rev. 2008 Apr 16;(2):CD001478
3. J Commun Dis. 2011 Sep;43(3):177-81
4. N Engl J Med. 1996 Feb 8;334(6):341-8
5. Med Hypotheses. 2010 Jan;74(1):150-4
6. Vaccine. 1993 Nov;11(14):1371-9
7. Pediatr Infect Dis J. 2004 Jun;23(6):568-71
8. Pediatr Int. 2004 Dec;46(6):650-5
9. not in use
10. BMJ. 1993 November 6; 307(6913): 1171–1176
11. Epidemiology. 1997 Nov;8(6):678-80
12. BMJ. 2004 April 17; 328(7445): 925–926
13. BMJ. 1993 November 6; 307(6913): 1171–1176
14. JAMA. 1994 Jan 5;271(1):37-41
15. Lancet. 1997 Nov 29;350(9091):1569-77

Prevnar 13

Manufacturer: Wyeth Pharmaceuticals, Inc (owned by Pfizer)
Generic name: Pneumococcal 13-valent Conjugate Vaccine (Diphtheria CRM197 Protein)

Prevnar 13 Safety

The manufacturer's clinical trials involved either administering Prevnar 13 with other vaccines at the same time or dividing subjects into one Prevnar 13 group and one Prevnar control group. In the first case it is impossible to know which vaccine caused a certain adverse event, allowing manufacturers to claim there is no evidence that it was their vaccine. In the second case there is no true placebo group, as both groups receive similar vaccines. Prevnar 13 was deemed to have a similar safety profile to Prevnar. Serious adverse events were said to be rare and included bronchiolitis, gastroenteritis and pneumonia (all recorded at 0.9%). The 3 sudden infant deaths recorded were said to be at no higher a rate than in the wider population. The longest follow-up period for serious adverse reactions was 30 days. [1]

The UK passive reporting system has recorded 21 deaths over 12 years possibly related to pneumococcal conjugate vaccines and the US system has recorded 1170 deaths over 13 years. Neither system tells us if the vaccine was really the cause but both also suffer from problems of under-reporting and the real figures could be much higher. The US fatality count is enormous whichever way one looks at it and should ring alarm bells. It constitutes a fifth of all deaths recorded on the VAERS database for all vaccines, ever.

Prevnar 13 Efficacy

The vaccine is designed to protect against 13 serotypes of the bacterium Streptococcus pneumonia, of which there are more than 90. It is not known what causes this common bacterium to become a pathogen.

Prevnar 13 efficacy was tested by showing that it was non-inferior to its predecessor (Prevnar) in terms of immunogenicity. Both vaccines caused comparable antibody responses and because Prevnar was considered effective, it was concluded that Prevnar 13 would be too. [1]

Turning then to Prevnar, the manufacturer refers to two main efficacy studies; one from California and one from Finland.

The Finnish study tried to establish whether Prevnar was effective in preventing otitis media (middle ear infection) in children. The results were moderate at best. The European regulator denied an application for the vaccine to be marketed as preventing otitis media (OM). In the US, on the other hand, the FDA was happy to agree that Prevnar could be marketed as preventing OM. Effectiveness was around 50% only where the illness was caused by a bacterial serotype that was contained in the vaccine. For other types there could even be a negative effectiveness, meaning that those vaccinated were more likely to get otitis media. [3] This hasn't prevented Wyeth/Pfizer from widely claiming its vaccines to be effective for preventing OM.

The California study looked at whether Prevnar prevented invasive disease caused by S. pneumoniae in general and involved over 37,000 children. The manufacturer says it was 100% effective. Sounds amazing! However, the reason for this perfect result was that Wyeth agreed with the US regulator (FDA) on 3rd November 1997 that they could stop the trial once 17 cases of invasive pneumococcal diseases had been recorded and as long as no more than 2 had occurred in the vaccine group. They could then claim efficacy and terminated the trial (all 17 were in fact recorded in the control group). [2] I'm concerned that such a selective approach leaves the results wide open to data manipulation. For example, over 7,000 subjects were excluded from the results for various reasons and although that in itself is not suspicious and may have been totally justified, it would be all to easy to "lose" a small number of cases from the vaccine group who did in fact get ill from pneumococcal infection, either deliberately or by mistake. Even the FDA had some concerns regarding the data but following requests of additional data from Wyeth, they were satisfied that the results were accurate.

The FDA did point out that the trial did not show whether the vaccine was effective for more than one year.

My conclusion is that if the results are accurate, then a protective benefit of only 12 months duration is not good enough and a long-lasting effect should have been established. I have no information that would disprove that the vaccine works for at least 12 months, but the way the trial was handled is certainly highly unsatisfactory, especially considering that the entire efficacy claim for the vaccine, its subsequent approval, and the approval of its successor Prevnar 13, all base on this one trial.

Prevnar 13 Adverse reactions (according to the manufacturer)

The following are taken from the manufacturers patient information leaflet. They will not include all side-effects and may not include the most serious ones.

- irritability (>70%)
- injection site tenderness (>50%)
- decreased appetite (>40%)
- decreased sleep (>40%)
- increased sleep (>40%)
- fever (>20%)
- injection site redness (>20%) and injection site swelling (>20%) (6.2)

Prevnar 13 Contraindications (according to the package insert)

Severe allergic reaction (e.g., anaphylaxis) to any component of Prevnar 13 or any diphtheria toxoid-containing vaccine

Ingredients

- 2mcg each of Streptococcus pneumoniae serotypes 1, 3, 4, 5, 6A, 7F, 9V, 14, 18C, 19A, 19F, 23F saccharides
- 4.4 mcg 6B saccharides
- 34 mcg CRM197 carrier protein
- 100 mcg Polysorbate 80 [can cause severe nonimmunologic anaphylactoid reactions]
- 295 mcg Succinate Buffer
- 125 mcg Aluminium Phosphate

References

1. Prevnar 13 prescribing information
2. Clinical Review of New Product License Application PLA 92-0279 – Prevnar
3. Clinical Review of Amendment to Product License Application

Priorix

Manufacturer: GlaxoSmithKline
Generic name: Measles, Mumps and Rubella vaccine (live)

Priorix Safety

GSK presented data which compared the rate of side-effects with another vaccine and according to those figures, Priorix caused most pre-determined adverse reactions less often than the other vaccine. Their product information does not state what the other vaccine was.

They also included "unsolicited events" (unlooked-for side-effects) but only for those subjects who completed the trial as per protocol. [1] This would have excluded any who dropped out exactly *because* of adverse reactions. But even with this little data manipulation, the results still make grim reading. Between 1 in 100 and 1 in 10 subjects suffered pharyngitis, bronchitis, upper respiratory tract infections, allergic reactions, vomiting, headaches, eczema, diarrhoea and otitis media. Fewer than 1 in 100 suffered dermatitis, herpes zoster, viral, bacterial or fungal infections, pneumonia, laryngitis, stridor, enteritis, gastroenteritis, anorexia, stomatitis, insomnia, anaemia, lymphadenopathy, granulocytopenia, exanthema, epididymitis, asthma, colitis, skin exfoliation and others. See below for additional adverse reactions.

In addition very serious adverse reactions have been observed since the vaccine was put into use but these are classed as very rare. I'm nevertheless reproducing them here because although they may be very rare, complications from measles, mumps and rubella are also very rare, which means parents may be exchanging very rare complications from the diseases for very rare side-effects from the vaccine. They include: athralgia and arthritis, anaphylactic reactions, meningitis, thrombocytopenia, thrombocytopenic purpura and erythema multiforme.

The vaccine can also cause symptoms which are very similar to those caused by the diseases it's meant to prevent, as well as the complications therefrom.[1]

The UK Yellow Card scheme has recorded over 8,000 reports and 28 deaths relating to MMR vaccines but this data covers a 27 year period and there is no certainty that the vaccines really caused these fatalities. Yet conversely, under-reporting means that the true incidence rate could be one hundred times higher.

9 out of the 38 fatalities were recorded simple as death, sudden death or sudden infant death. It is not unreasonable to suggest that the vast majority of SIDs will never be reported as vaccine related, even if they happened soon after vaccination.

On the US VAERS database, MMR vaccines make up 15% of the entire database of adverse reactions. Most of them were classed as "not serious". 324 were for deaths and over 1000 each for "life threatening" or "permanent disability". Once again this data does not prove that vaccines were responsible in all cases but neither does it reflect the true number of cases due to under-reporting. It only tells us that MMR vaccines are one of the most reported vaccine types on the database.

Priorix Efficacy

From the data presented in the manufacturer's product information, it appears that Priorix has only been tested for immunogenicity and that no protectiveness field trial has been conducted. GSK measured antibody density in trial subjects for up to one year following vaccination and found that almost everyone had the looked-for antibody reaction, something which applies to most vaccines. The crux of whether this means a child is protected was not examined but is assumed to be the case.

Whether this is reasonable or not is arguable. The immunogenicity = protection axiom is widely accepted in medicine and if it is true, then the vaccine will protect children for at least a year. However, plenty of cases are known where diseases broke out in populations where almost everyone was adequately vaccinated and where, consequently, the vaccine did not protect these children. Examples are listed in the relevant chapters for Measles Mumps and Rubella. I have also discussed the issue of waning immunity from vaccines on those pages where relevant.

Priorix Contraindications (according to the package insert)

Priorix should not be given
- if you or your child is allergic against any of the components of this vaccine. Signs of an allergic reaction may include itchy skin rash, shortness of breath and swelling of the face or tongue;
- if you or your child is known to be allergic to neomycin (an antibiotic agent). A known contact dermatitis (skin rash when the skin is in direct contact with allergens such as neomycin) should not be a prblem but talk to your doctor first;
- if you or your child has a severe infection with a high temperature. In these cases, the vaccination will be postponed until recovery. A minor infection such as a cold should not be a problem, but talk to your doctor first;
- if you or your child has any illness (such as Human Immunodeficiency Virus (HIV) or Acquired Immunodeficiency Syndrome (AIDS)) or takes any medicine that weakens the immune system. Whether you or your child receives the vaccine will depend upon the level of your immune defences.
- if you or your child is pregnant. In addition, pregnancy should be avoided for 1 month following vaccination.

Warnings and precautions
Talk to your doctor or pharmacist before you or your child receives Priorix:
- if you or your child has disorders of the central nervous system, a history of convulsion accompanying high fever or family history of convulsions. In case of high fever following vaccination please consult your doctor promptly;
- if you or your child has ever had a severe allergic reaction to egg protein;
- if you or your child has had a side effect after vaccination against measles, mumps or rubella that involved easy bruising or bleeding for longer than usual;

• if you or your child has weakened immune system (e.g. such as HIV infection). You or your child should be closely monitored as the responses to the vaccines may not be sufficient to ensure a protection against the illness.

Priorix Adverse Reactions/Side-effects (according to the package insert)

Side effects that occurred during clinical trials with Priorix were as follows:

Very common (these may occur with more than 1 in 10 doses of the vaccine):
• redness at the injection site
• fever of 38°C or higher

Common (these may occur with up to 1 in 10 doses of the vaccine):
• Pain and swelling at the injection site
• fever higher than 39.5°C
• rash (spots)
• upper respiratory tract infection

Uncommon (these may occur with up to 1 in 100 doses of the vaccine):
• infection of the middle ear
• swollen lymph glands (glands in the neck, armpit or groin)
• loss of appetite
• nervousness
• abnormal crying
• inability to sleep (insomnia)
• redness, irritation and watering of the eyes (conjunctivitis)
• bronchitis
• cough
• swollen parotid glands (glands in the cheek)
• diarrhoea
• vomiting

Rare (these may occur with up to 1 in 1,000 doses of the vaccine):
• convulsions accompanying high fever
• allergic reactions

After the marketing of Priorix, the following additional side effects have been reported on a few occasions:

• joint pain and inflammation
• punctual or small spotted bleeding or bruising more easily than normal due to a drop in platelets
• sudden life-threatening allergic reaction
• inflammation of the meninges, brain, spinal cord and peripheral nerves, Guillain-Barré syndrome (ascending paralysis up to respiratory paralysis)

- Kawasaki syndrome (major signs of the illness are for instance: fever, skin rash, swollen lymph glands, inflammation and rash of the mucous membranes of the mouth and throat)
- Erythema multiforme (symptoms are red, often itchy spots, similar to the rash of measles, which starts on the limbs and sometimes on the face and the rest of the body).
- Measles and mumps like symptoms
- reduced measles
- transient, painful swelling of the testicles

Ingredients

The active substances are:
- measles, mumps and rubella live attenuated viruses

The other ingredients are:

- amino acids
- lactose (anhydrous)
- mannitol
- sorbitol
- water for injections

References
1. Priorix product information

Repevax

Manufacturer: Sanofi Pasteur MSD
Generic name: Diphtheria, Tetanus, Pertussis (acellular, component) and Poliomyelitis (inactivated) Vaccine (adsorbed, reduced antigen content)

Repevax Safety

I have only been able to find very scant information about safety trials for Repevax. The manufacturer only disclosed that 390 children aged 3-6 received Repevax as a pre-school booster and that the side-effects listed further below in this chapter were found. Neither the UK, European nor US regulators had published any further information at the time of writing.

The vaccine should not be used in pregnancy and is not meant to be used for primary immunisation.

Repevax Efficacy

The efficacy claim bases on immunogenicity/antibody response and the manufacturer says that almost everyone who received the vaccine as a booster developed the looked-for antibody levels when measured one month later. They also say they conducted a follow-up study which found that antibody levels were maintained after 5 years. No efficacy trial was done in the sense of finding out if vaccinated children are protected from illness but Sanofi Pasteur refers to a Swedish trial that showed protectiveness for a similar vaccine. This Swedish trial only looked into the Pertussis part of the vaccine and compared the protective effects of different pertussis vaccines against each other. There was no real placebo group.

Whether the vaccine is effective or not therefore depends on whether immunogenicity really equals protection. Some studies suggest it does while others suggest it doesn't.

Further detail can be found in the relevant chapters for Diphtheria, Tetanus, Pertussis and Polio.

Repevax Contraindications (according to the manufacturer)

REPEVAX should not be administered to persons with known hypersensitivity
• to diphtheria, tetanus, pertussis or poliomyelitis vaccines
• to any other component of the vaccine (see Section 6.1)
• to any residual substances carried over from manufacture (formaldehyde, glutaraldehyde, streptomycin, neomycin, polymyxin B and bovine serum albumin), which may be present in undetectable trace amounts.

REPEVAX should not be administered to persons who experienced an encephalopathy of unknown origin within 7 days of previous immunization with a pertussis-containing vaccine.

As with other vaccines, administration of REPEVAX should be postponed in persons suffering from an acute severe febrile illness. The presence of a minor infection (e.g., mild upper respiratory infection) is not a contraindication.

Repevax Adverse Events / Side-effects (according to the manufacturer)

Very common (more than 1 in 10)
• Fatigue
• Fever
• Irritability
• Pain Swelling
• Erythema

Common (1 in 100 to 1 in 10)
• Headache
• Diarrhoea
• Vomiting
• Nausea
• Rash
• Athralgia
• Joint Swelling
• Dermatitis
• Bruising
• Pruritus

Unknown Frequency
• Lymphadenopathy
• Anaphylactic reactions
• Convulsions
• Vasovagal Syncope
• Guillain Barré syndrome
• Facial Palsy
• Myelitis
• Brachial Neuritis
• Transient paresthesia/hypoesthesia of vaccinated limb
• Dizziness
• Malaise
• Pallor
• Extensive limb swelling
• Injection site induration

(the frequency listed here is that which was found in children)

Ingredients

- Diphtheria toxoid
- Tetanus toxoid
- Pertussis antigens
- Perussis toxoid
- Filamentous Haemagglutinin
- Pertactin
- Fimbriae Types 2 and 3
- Poliovirus (inactivated, produced in vero cells) Type 1-3

REPEVAX may contain traces of formaldehyde, glutaraldehyde, streptomycin, neomycin, polymyxin B and bovine serum albumin, which are used during the manufacturing process.

Repevax also contains: Phenoxyethanol, Polysorbate 80, water for injections

Revaxis

Manufacturer: Sanofi Pasteur MSD
Generic name: Diphtheria, tetanus and poliomyelitis (inactivated) vaccine (adsorbed, reduced antigen(s) content)

Revaxis Safety

Information publicly available for Revaxis is limited. The manufacturer states that the adverse reactions listed further below were found in clinical trials but gives no further detail. None of the regulators have published any further information. I'm therefore not in a position to evaluate the studies at this time.

Revaxis Efficacy

Sanofi Pasteur says that the vaccine produced good antibody responses in clinical trials and that these were still evident after 2 years follow-up. There is no mention of a proper efficacy trial but as usual, immunogenicity is assumed to be the same as immunity.
Due to the limited information published for Revaxis, I cannot evaluate its efficacy further at this time.

Contraindications according to the manufacturer

Do not use Revaxis if you or your child:

• is allergic (hypersensitive) to
    ~ the active substances of Revaxis
    ~ any of the other ingredients
    ~ neomycin, streptomycin or polymyxin B which can be present
      in trace amounts
• has ever had an allergic reaction to any vaccine for diphtheria, tetanus or
  polio
• has ever had any neurological problems (such as weakness or numbness)
  after a previous injection of a vaccine against diphtheria or tetanus.
• has an acute severe illness (infection) with a high temperature. The vaccination will be delayed until you/your child has recovered. A minor infection is not usually a reason to postpone vaccination. Your doctor or nurse will decide if you or your child should receive the vaccine.

Take special care with Revaxis
Tell your doctor or nurse before vaccination if you or your child:

• has a blood disorder where you or your child bruise or bleed easily (such as haemophilia or thrombocytopenia).

- has ever had a temporary loss of movement and feeling in all or part of the body or loss of movement, pain and numbness of the arm and the shoulder after having a vaccine which contains tetanus (Guillain-Barré syndrome or brachial neuritis).
- has had a vaccine for diphtheria or tetanus within the last 5 years. Your doctor will decide on the basis of local recommendations whether you or your child can receive a further injection or not.
- has a poor or reduced immune system, because of a course of medical treatment (e.g., steroids, chemotherapy or radiotherapy), HIV infection or any other illness.

The vaccine may not protect as well as it protects people with normal immune systems. The vaccination may be postponed until your/your child's immune system has recovered.

Adverse Reactions/Side-effects according to the manufacturer

Serious allergic reactions
These reactions are always a rare possibility after receiving a vaccine and may include:
- difficulty in breathing
- blue discolouration of the tongue or lips
- swelling of the face or throat
- low blood pressure (causing dizziness)
- fainting (collapse)

During clinical studies, the following side effects were observed:
Very common side effects (reported in more than 1 out of 10 people):
- local reactions at the site of injection: pain, redness, hardening of the skin (induration), swelling or nodule.
Common side effects (reported by less than 1 in 10 people):
- dizziness (vertigo)
- feeling sick and being sick (nausea and vomiting)
- a high temperature (fever)
- headache
Uncommon side effects (reported by less than 1 in 100 people):
- swollen glands (lymphadenopathy)
- feeling generally unwell (malaise)
- muscle pains (myalgia)
Rare side effects (reported by less than 1 in 1,000 people):
- joint pains (arthralgia)

Additionally, the following side effects have been reported very rarely during the commercial use of Revaxis; however, exact incidence rates cannot be precisely calculated:
- pain in the vaccinated limb
- large reactions at the injection site (larger than 5 cm), including extensive limb swelling from the injection site beyond one or both joints
- uncontrollable shivering (chills) and flu-like symptoms
- feeling weak and looking pale (asthenia, pallor)
- abdominal pain, diarrhoea

- allergic reactions such as hives or skin rash, swelling of the face (facial oedema)
- serious allergic reactions including shock (anaphylactic reactions including shock)
- fainting (vasovagal syncope)
- 'pins and needles' or numbness in the vaccinated limb (transient paresthesia and hypoesthesia)
- temporary loss of movement or feeling (Guillain-Barré syndrome); loss of movement, pain and numbness of the arm and the shoulder (brachial neuritis); convulsions

Ingredients

- Purified Diphtheria Toxoid
- Purified Tetanus Toxoid
- Inactivated Poliomyelitis virus (produced in Vero cells)
- aluminium hydroxide
- phenoxyethanol
- formaldehyde
- Medium 199 (a mixture of amino acids including phenylalanine, mineral salts, vitamins, polysorbate 80 and other substances)
- water for injections.

Rotarix

Manufacturer: GlaxoSmithKline
Generic name: Rotavirus Vaccine, Live, Oral

Rotarix Safety

Side-effects were investigated in several clinical trials where Rotarix was compared to a placebo group. In some trials, both groups also received other vaccines at the same time. Neither GSK nor the regulator say whether the placebo was a true placebo or another vaccine. A real placebo is sometimes called a saline placebo, but here only a "placebo" is mentioned. As this term has often been used to mean another vaccine or a substance containing the non-active ingredients of the trial vaccine, we cannot be sure which is the case.

The clinical trials found no increased risk for adverse reactions from Rotarix. Serious adverse reactions were all judged to be not vaccine related by GSK's study investigators.[1]

The US VAERS database has recorded up to 20 deaths, 41 life-threatening events and 291 hospitalisations per year possibly due to live rotavirus oral vaccines. Although VAERS staff follow up all serious reports, the data does not mean that the vaccine was to blame for all or even any of the cases. At the same time, vaccine adverse reactions are thought to be widely under-reported and the reported numbers could reflect as little as 1% of cases.

Parents should be aware that the virus contained in the vaccine can be shed in infants' stool and infect other household members.

Rotarix Efficacy

Unlike some other vaccines, Rotarix underwent proper efficacy trials. Rather then looking at immunogenicity only, these trials examined how many children got ill from severe rotavirus gastroenteritis during a certain time period following vaccination. In the main study conducted in Latin America, several thousand children received the vaccine or a placebo and during an average follow-up time of 8 months, subjects in the vaccine group were much less likely to get ill from severe rotavirus gastroenteritis and the vaccine was found to be 85% effective. A year later the vaccines effectiveness was still calculated at 79%, although the regulator found this figure unreliable.

In a similar study in Finland, the vaccine effectiveness was found to be 72-90% but I'm not aware how long the follow-up period was. In another study the effectiveness was 55%-93% but again I'm unaware of the follow-up period.
The results depend on various factors, such as what serotype of the virus caused the disease and whether protectiveness was measured against all incidents or only severe ones etc.

As the European Medicines Agency points out in its assessments, the overall incidence rate was low. The rate of infants who got ill was under 1% even in the placebo groups. The EMA raised a number of concerns over how the data was compiled and presented, including a change in outcome definition in the largest study. However, further responses from GSK were satisfactory to the EMA.

The EMA also pointed out that infants still have maternal antibodies in their blood at the age of vaccination but they were satisfied that the studies had adequately taken this into consideration.[1]

I would have been interested to learn how many children got ill from non-rotavirus gastroenteritis in those trials. Although the vaccine can't be expected to protect against these, it would have shown what impact vaccinating against rotavirus has overall, especially as so few infants got ill from rotavirus.

Side-effects/adverse reactions (according to the package insert)

GlaxoSmithKline's information on adverse reactions says that the following occurred as much in the placebo group as it did in the Rotarix group during trials:

irritability (52%), cough/runny nose (around 25-30%), fever (around 25%), loss of appetite (around 25%), vomiting (around 12%) and diarrhea (around 4%).

GSK say that serious adverse events happened more often in the placebo group than in the Rotarix group, including gastroenteritis, diarrhea and dehydration.

They also say that 0.19% of the Rotarix trial group and 0.15% of the placebo group died following administration.

Contraindication according to the package insert)

Hypersensitivity

A demonstrated history of hypersensitivity to any component of the vaccine.

Infants who develop symptoms suggestive of hypersensitivity after receiving a dose of ROTARIX should not receive further doses of ROTARIX.

Gastrointestinal Tract Congenital Malformation

Infants with a history of uncorrected congenital malformation of the gastrointestinal tract (such as Meckel's diverticulum) that would predispose the infant for intussusception should not receive ROTARIX.

History of Intussusception

Infants with a history of intussusception should not receive ROTARIX. In postmarketing experience, intussusception resulting in death following a second dose has been reported following a history of intussusception after the first dose.

Severe Combined Immunodeficiency Disease

Infants with Severe Combined Immunodeficiency Disease (SCID) should not receive ROTARIX. Postmarketing reports of gastroenteritis, including severe diarrhea and prolonged shedding of vaccine virus, have been reported in infants who were administered live, oral rotavirus vaccines and later identified as having SCID.

Ingredients

- Human rotavirus RIX4414 strain (live, attenuated) produced on vero cells
- Sucrose
- Di-sodium Adipate
- Dulbecco's Modified Eagle Medium (DMEM): amino acids, calcium chloride, potassium chloride, magnesium sulfate, sodium chloride, monosodium phosphate, glucose, vitamins, iron, phenol red
- Sterile water

References

1. European Medicines Agency Scientific Discussion papers 2006

Printed in Great Britain
by Amazon